SCALES
TO
SCALPELS

DOCTORS WHO PRACTICE THE HEALING
ARTS OF MUSIC AND MEDICINE

DR. LISA WONG

WITH ROBERT VIAGAS

PEGASUS BOOKS
NEW YORK

SCALES TO SCALPELS

Pegasus Books LLC
80 Broad Street, 5th Floor
New York, NY 10004

Interior design by Maria Fernandez

ISBN: 978-1-60598-177-2

10 9 8 7 6 5 4 3 2 1

Printed in the United States of America
Distributed by W. W. Norton & Company, Inc.

For the musicians and the audiences

of the Longwood Symphony Orchestra,

and to all medical musicians around the world who

are inspired by the guiding spirit and profound

example of Dr. Albert Schweitzer.

I am so grateful to my husband Lynn and my inspirational musical children, Jennifer and Christopher, for their warmth, encouragement and unbridled love. Additional thanks go to my extended family: to my parents who supported and encouraged me to pursue each of my passions; to my in-laws, who were my medical role models; and to my siblings whose playfulness and curiosity made music fun throughout our childhood.

Thanks to Robert Viagas for pursuing this journey with me and to my many friends who contributed their keen eyes, sympathetic ears and comforting shoulders.

—Lisa Wong

I thank my sons, Ben and Nick, who are my motivation and inspiration. I thank my friends who stood by my side and kept me going through a tough year. And I thank the remarkable musicians of the Longwood Symphony Orchestra, who were generous enough to let me peek over their shoulders while they did their amazing work.

—Robert Viagas

CONTENTS

Foreword

by Bernard Lown, M.D.

Just as my fingers on these keys
Make music, so the self-same sounds
On my spirit make a music, too.
Music is feeling, then, not sound.

Wallace Stevens

THE OLDER I GROW, THE more convinced I become that the miracle of life is that miracles do happen. For example, this very book, *Scales to Scalpels,* is a tale of the miraculous that awes the reader with a profound insight: when people devote their lives not merely to the quest for self-fulfillment but also to a communal quest for worthiness, the miraculous is close at hand.

How else to explain the phenomenon—nay, the miracle— of the Longwood Symphony Orchestra (LSO), a volunteer group of more than one hundred health professionals who have been performing classical concerts for nearly thirty years. These are overachievers whose every moment is at a premium, who continuously forage scarce time in pursuit of medical and musical excellence. They perform without fiscal reward, without much personal recognition, investing hours in rehearsal as they aim for an elusive musical perfection. The musicians share each performance with a healthcare or community organization that responds to the needs of the underserved, the abandoned, and the forgotten. Every concert thus makes an enduring difference. The music-making is not limited to orchestral performances: the LSO also offers on a monthly basis outreach programs featuring small ensembles that play in senior centers, hospices, rehabilitation centers, homeless shelters, and hospitals.

A puzzling fact is the special affinity between scientifically trained health professionals and classical-music making. *Scales to Scalpels* probes this phenomenon and offers a bevy of theories and persuasive explanations. As a medical practitioner of fifty-five years, I have been increasingly discomfited by the tension between science and the arts that characterizes modern medicine. Science, in the form of innovative technologies, increasingly views the patient as an amalgam of dysfunctional parts, while the arts, since time immemorial, have probed the meaning of being human. The former focuses on curing a disease; the latter aims to heal a human being brimming with uncertainty, discomfort, and dread.

Science is constantly providing new and ever more powerful tools. Current imaging techniques leave no part of the body unexposed. None of these, however, can reveal the basis of an aching heart. This is left to the art of medicine, which has remained largely unchanged over millennia. Its most powerful tool is listening to a patient's words. But language is a grossly imperfect tool for communicating the tonalities of being, let alone conveying the disruptions imposed by illness. As Gustave Flaubert lamented in his magisterial novel, *Madame Bovary:* "None of us can ever express the exact measure of his needs or his thoughts or his sorrows; and human speech is like a cracked kettle on which we tap crude rhythms for bears to dance to, while we long to make music that will melt the stars." Of all the science that a physician acquires, of all the skills mastered, listening is by far the most difficult. This seemingly simple act requires consummate artistry. Listening, like musical virtuosity, demands intense cultivation. To the ancient Sumerians the word for *ear* and *wisdom* was the same. Proper listening enables one to comprehend the unique narrative of another human being. Even at its scientific best, medicine is dependent on the intimate story. For doctors, listening is an exhilarating act of discovery; for patients, it identifies a healer.

Doctors nowadays are far more stressed as they increasingly become the tools of their tools. Less time is spent listening to patients. Human connections are frayed. Trust is undermined. Patients surf the Internet and visit multiple specialists to gain relief for what ails them. Doctors realize something is missing in their lives. Those blessed with musical talent find in performing a new venue for listening. Orchestral cohesion and enhanced musicality demand listening intimately to fellow musicians. Only when they are tuned to one another do they achieve tonalities that can "melt the stars."

The LSO is more than an orchestra. It is a community organizer. By bringing music to the most needy, it not only heals what ails people physically but also fills a spiritual void. To the alienated in the rough and tumble of urban anarchy, the LSO serves as a role model of how the meaning of existence is nurtured by serving others. As the consummate physician essayist Lewis Thomas wrote in *Late Night Thoughts on Listening to Mahler's Ninth Symphony,* "I am inclined to assert unconditionally, that there is one central, universal aspect of human behavior, genetically set by our very nature, biologically governed, driving each of us along. ... it can be defined as the urge to be useful. This urge drives society along, sets our behavior as individuals and in groups, invents all our myths, writes our poetry, composes our music."

In coupling music-making with communal engagement, the LSO is following in the footsteps of Dr. Albert Schweitzer, humanist, physician, musician, and scholar. Schweitzer expressed his reverence for life by doctoring those living in Lambaréné, Gabon. The modern-day troubadours of the LSO, by melding music with healing, foster emotional connectivity and spirituality in the cathedral of our turbulent urban space.

Bernard Lown, M.D.
Professor Harvard School of Public Health
Senior Physician Emeritus Brigham
and Women's Hospital, Boston

Foreword

by Dr. Lisa Wong

I HAVE SPENT MY LIFE sharing the healing arts of music and medicine with patients and audiences. Contrary to what you might think, there are strong parallels between the two. Both require high degrees of training, passion, focus, and the sharing of humanity. When a musician looks at a piece of music, the notes are just dots on a page—a visual representation of an aural experience. Once analyzed, digested, and understood, and once the musician adds his or her own voice, experience and creativity, those dots can miraculously transform into wrenchingly beautiful or heartbreakingly passionate music. As doctors, we similarly see that a medical diagnosis can come strictly from set of lab tests or stack of X-rays. Medicine is as much an art as music: we incorporate knowledge of anatomy and physiology, add experience, and creativity—and arrive at an elegant diagnosis that is unique to the patient. Just as we listen to the music, we must listen to the patient.

Healing the community through music is a shared belief in my own family. My husband, violinist Lynn Chang, the eldest son of two doctors, might have become a doctor had he not won the 1974 International Paganini Competition in Italy while still a Harvard undergraduate. When he returned to Cambridge, he happily withdrew from organic chemistry (although I think he would have made a fine doctor!) to become a professional musician. He cares for people through his music; as a performer and teacher, he has mentored and encouraged scores of young people to follow their journeys and pursue their dreams, musical or not. Some of his students have found places in America's top orchestras, from Los Angeles to Chicago to Boston. Others have continued their music while working as physicians, engineers or scientists. We share the belief that music touches lives and effects true social change. Last December, Lynn was invited to perform at the 2010 Nobel Peace Prize ceremony for poet Liu Xiaobo, an imprisoned human rights advocate. There, performing to a symbolically empty chair, Lynn's music spoke powerfully. Hans Christian Anderson's oft-quoted phrase rang true: "Where words fail, music speaks."

This book traces the lives of several of my musical and medical colleagues who are equally devoted to changing the world through their medicine and music. This is the story of the Longwood Symphony Orchestra, Boston's ensemble of medical professionals. Just as each instrument plays a different role in a symphony so each member of the LSO plays a unique role in this medical musical ensemble. Some are powerhouse young students at the beginning of their journeys. Others are elder statesmen physicians with years of orchestra experience behind them. For twenty-eight years, the orchestra has done its part to make the world a better, healthier and more melodic place by balancing three equal elements—music, medicine and community service.

We have devoted our lives to healing our community. Over the past century, medical discoveries and technology have eradicated many diseases, improved quality of life, and increased life expectancy. But there are limits to what medical technology can do. As doctors, we need to return our medical roots. Often, a diagnosis is made not by another lab test or CAT scan but by sitting quietly with our patient. A person's "vital signs" go beyond temperature and blood pressure to temperament and emotion. Our musical training helps us to listen, not just hear, and to recognize that there is a song in every diagnosis.

Dr. Lisa Wong
Boston, November 2011

SCALES

TO

SCALPELS

PART I

INTRODUCING THE MUSICIAN-PHYSICIAN

1

Overture to the Musician-Physician

CHANCES ARE, YOUR DOCTOR HAS a secret life.

As a musician.

When the patients all go home, the old magazines in the waiting room are stacked back into a neat pile, blood-pressure cuffs put away, and assorted medical instruments bathed in their disinfectant, many doctors then take out their *other* instruments—violins, violas, flutes, bassoons, cellos, contrabasses, tubas, French horns, oboes d'amore. . . . And they make joyful noise. Talk about a secret life! But the two sides of their personalities are more closely linked than you'd think. A burst of recent research is showing that music itself is a kind of medicine, a toning and a tonic for both the body and the mind.

I'm Dr. Lisa M. Wong, and I'd like to introduce you to an organization that has been a part of my life for over twenty years. As president of the remarkable Longwood Symphony orchestra, an all-volunteer ensemble consisting almost entirely of doctors and other health care professionals who, like me, are driven to play music. I'd like to take you by the hand and take you inside the lives of my colleagues who have two—and sometimes three or four—amazing skills. They use music to heal their patients, heal their community, and, often, heal themselves as well. They are part of the fascinating, growing awareness of the interplay between music and medicine. I'd like to take you backstage and show you the issues, people, research, and stories surrounding our orchestra and what we do.

DR. KIMBERLY'S RIDE

When talking about the Longwood Symphony Orchestra, it all starts with our musicians. So let me introduce Dr. Heidi Harbison Kimberly, an emergency room doctor at Brigham and Women's Hospital here in Boston. Tall, slender, and muscular, with glasses magnifying her blue eyes, she has shoulder-length brown hair usually pinned up casually on the back of her head. She sits near me in the violin section where we meet every week.

Let's look over her shoulder as she is ending her shift late on the evening of a rehearsal.

She finishes stabilizing a trauma patient who barely survived a car accident. When she sees the patient is safely on the way to Intensive Care, Dr. Kimberly yanks her violin case from where she has stashed it under a desk. Colleagues used to ask her what it was—a 1930s Chicago mobster named Sebastiano Domingo apparently really did carry his machine gun in a violin case—but by now they're accustomed to her routine. She slings the violin case over her shoulders like a pack and dashes out to the rack where her bright red mountain bike stands waiting. She snaps off the u-lock, jams on her helmet, slips on ankle reflectors and switches on flashing safety lights, then leaps aboard and begins pedaling nimbly down the narrow street behind the hospital. Because of her position hunched over the handlebars, the violin rides up behind her head, pressing on her helmet and forcing her to crane her neck to see her way.

Her ride, a five-minute slalom through some of the top hospitals in the world, takes her backward through her career. Leaving the hospital where she works (and where she trained), she passes the hospital where she did her residency, then cuts through the quad of the Harvard Medical School, where she earned her medical degree. Ring-ringing the bell on her handlebars, she threads her way through the traffic and crowds on Longwood Avenue itself, then skids to a stop in front of the venerable Boston Latin School, where our orchestra rehearses. She's been riding this same route to rehearsal for the past eleven years. It's like the midnight ride of Paul Revere—which actually occurred only a few miles from Longwood Avenue with a much earlier Bostonian—except it's "the musicians are coming, the musicians are coming."

Parts of the Boston Latin School, founded in 1635, were already standing when Revere made his famous ride to warn of the British invasion. Dr. Kimberly patters up the steps into a hallway filled with her medical colleagues pulling their own musical instruments out of their cases and playing trills and arpeggios to warm up. It's very social. "How are things going? How was your vacation? Did you finish your surgical rotation? How were the Boards?"

"It's like a social parade into rehearsal," Kimberly said. "Finally someone starts clapping and yelling, 'C'mon everybody! Let's get going! Time for rehearsal!' And herding people in. I'm one of the ones who have to be herded."

However venerable its origins, the Boston Latin School band room looks pretty much the same as any high school band room. There's the same after-hours cleaning fluid smell, the same acoustic walls, the same lockers for instruments. Down the hall, the custodians are playing easy rock from their radios as they work, but over time have come to love our hearing our rehearsals so much that they have also become regulars at our concerts. Inside the band room, fresh young medical students alongside revered elder doctor specialists lend a shoulder to push aside pianos and drum sets to make room for their folding chairs and music stands. There's no air-conditioning, and the room becomes a sauna on summer days. Dr. Kimberly wipes her brow, swipes rosin on her bow, and arranges pages of music for herself and her stand partner.

Waiting on his podium is our conductor, Maestro Jonathan McPhee, erect and trim with grave blue eyes, swept-back dark hair, and salt-and-pepper beard. Put him in a commodore's hat and you'd think he could command a flotilla—which, in a way, he does. During his six years with the orchestra, he can be credited with raising the playing quality and diversifying the repertoire, and he commands respect from this band of perfectionists. Standing square-shouldered and calm, he waits for quiet.

Here before him is the Longwood Symphony Orchestra. They range from Type A personalities to Type AAA. Someone once compared McPhee's job to herding cats, but sometimes it seems more like herding pumas. Ambitious, driven, successful—and sometimes neurotic—pumas. McPhee makes an announcement or two, congratulates one member on a prestigious grant, another who is headed to Europe on a fellowship, yet another on a newly completed second or third doctorate, and announces the first piece to be rehearsed.

Dr. Kimberly, her odyssey from the ICU completed, tucks her violin under her chin and raises her bow. Without another wasted moment, the conductor raises his baton and begins.

MANY MIRACLES

I'm there too at every rehearsal, sitting in the violin or viola section. In my other life, I'm a pediatrician at Milton Pediatric Associates, a thriving practice south of Boston where I've worked for over twenty-five years. Helping children navigate through life in a healthy way is my passion, and I've been lucky enough to do it in association with talented colleagues at nearly every hospital on Longwood Avenue. Having heard about this unique medical orchestra through other musician-physicians, I joined the LSO in 1985, took a seat on the Board of Directors in 1987, and was elected president in 1991.

In my work as a doctor, I witness many miracles. In my work as a musician, I count the weekly music-making in the LSO to be equally miraculous. I've watched my musical colleagues, all remarkable people who do remarkable work and remarkable research—still find the time—still *make* the time—to create this remarkable music. By day, our musicians take their place in clinics, hospitals, and medical schools as internists, surgeons, oncologists, cardiologists, psychologists, pediatricians, and more. By night, they are serious, devoted musicians. They do it not for their own personal gain, but for the love of the music, the camaraderie and love of the symphonic art form, which brings more than a hundred disparate personalities and their instruments performing together in harmony. We're not alone. The Longwood Symphony Orchestra is just one of more than a dozen other medical orchestras in the U.S. And, to answer your first question, we *do* allow beepers to go off during rehearsals, but never during performances!

We play for an even more compelling reason—to raise awareness and support for medically-related charities in Boston. For twenty years, the Longwood Symphony Orchestra has its own unique way of collaborating and fundraising for these charities, which I'll discuss in more detail in future chapters. Over the years we have worked with organizations addressing such public health issues as domestic violence, homelessness, and hunger, supporting patients with cancer, hemophilia, and diabetes, to name just a few.

Why do we do it? Playing music is another way for us to heal. This book will break down the question into parts and, I hope, offer a few answers. But it's a tricky proposition. When you reach out your hand and try to touch the place between medicine and music, some place between the physical and the spiritual, you're coming close to one of the fundamental mysteries of life. It delves close to the core of what makes us human.

MEDICAL MAIN STREET

The Longwood Symphony Orchestra takes its name from Longwood Avenue—the main street of the Boston medical district where many of our players have their "day jobs": Beth Israel Deaconess Medical Center, Children's Hospital Boston, Brigham and Women's Hospital, the Dana-Farber Cancer Institute, and, as the street's centerpiece, the marble acropolis of the Harvard Medical School. Medical facilities of one kind or another have stood on this site since colonial days.

This street is the Broadway of Boston's medical community, and home turf to many of the musicians in the LSO. It's not a wide street, but, apart from a grassy mall where the Harvard buildings cluster, it's intensely developed in a jumble of old and new architectural styles. You can tell that some of these institutions have been here more than a century because there is often a classic-looking stone building with a newer concrete extension and then an even newer glass extension. And many building sport scaffolding and warning signs indicating that yet another expansion is underway. Longwood Avenue is a work perpetually in progress. New techniques, new technology, and new treatments mean new wings.

The hundreds of doctors who work on this street can't help but see themselves as part of a medical tradition that began long before they got here and is certain to continue long after they are gone. It's the same with the classical music we play. We are privileged to be a part of the ongoing musical tradition and do our part to keep it healthy and give it a long life. We are working and playing to ensure that both are here for future generations.

We combine two ancient archetypes: the healer and the troubadour. Perhaps at one point in the distant past they were the same thing: a traveling shaman who would play a rudimentary instrument, chant and use mysterious herbs and unguents to ease the suffering of our distant ancestors, or even to cure them. Perhaps that is why some of us are here today. The musicians of the LSO have found a way to bring both traditions into counterpoint.

Of the one hundred and twenty member musicians of the Longwood Symphony Orchestra, we use ninety in a typical concert. With our medical and scientific obligations, not everyone can make every concert and we have backups for each section. In this book you'll meet, among others, an occupational therapist who helped bring a patient back from a coma-like state with music, an emergency room physician who dashes from the ER to the concert hall, cancer patients who lessen pain and depression with melody, and a pediatric surgeon who shakes off tension by picking up her violin.

Many of us have "crossover" stories. One violinist's medical school professor shared a music stand with her in the second violin section. A cellist was appointed chief resident for the bassoonist's medical team. And it isn't unusual for sage advice to be shared by an old hand with the student cramming for a physiology exam during the rests. Or for curbside medical consults to happen during rehearsal breaks. Abdominal pain? don't ask the violinist—he's a dermatologist. Better to seek the advice of the bassoonist, one of the best gastroenterologists in town.

These are people who touch your heart—in a few cases, literally.

"Plays" Well With Others
Both music and medicine engage the mind at its highest level. Performing with others and caring for patients in

a team requires similar multi-sensory training. Ensemble musicians are making multiple high-level decisions at every moment—decisions about rhythm, pitch, harmony, tempo—constantly adjusting to who is playing and what is going on around them. Physicians, too, are making decisions about the intonation of the body, the rhythm of the heart, the pitch, harmony, and tempo of a patient's life. Both endeavors require emotional intelligence and close collaboration in order to achieve success. They demand focus, intent listening, and communication. When you're playing in a chamber ensemble or treating a patient, there can be no success without a key ingredient: empathy. Our hearts reach out for the feelings of others, whether we are trying to harmonize with a fellow musician or trying to understand the source of a patient's pain.

Dr. Kimberly is a case in point. Growing up in Springfield, Massachusetts, she reminisces about a home full of music. Her father is a cardiologist and violist and her mother is a violinist. One of her earliest memories is falling asleep to the sounds of her mother's chamber group practicing downstairs. Even today, whenever she gets together with her parents, they make time to play trios.

"My mother wanted to make music fun," she said. "And she believed that to do that, you had to play with others. Throughout my life I've seen again and again how right she was. Playing violin not only makes me a happier, more well-rounded person, I believe it makes me a better physician, better able to take care of people.

"I took a course in medical school called 'Living With Life-Threatening Illness.' They pair you with actual oncology patients who have terminal cancer and you're supposed to meet with them every week. I was paired with a woman named Judy who had ovarian cancer. We really hit it off and a big part of that was because she loved music. She told me she loved the music of Bohuslav Martinu, and I thought that was so amazing because Martinu is not a commonly known composer. She said she liked his music because it was so happy and joyful. Whenever she went to the hospital—which sadly became more and more frequently—she always brought music.

"At the end of the course, we were supposed to stop seeing the patients, but Judy and I kept in touch and even went to concerts together. They later asked me to speak at her memorial service. I wrote a letter to her family saying how she changed my life in medicine. I said I admired the way she confronted her illness. She wasn't sad or angry or bitter. She accepted that death was coming and decided to do things that made her happy. She liked to make ceramics, go to the beach—and listen to music. At the end of her life when she was confined to the hospital, she couldn't do those other things. But she was still listening to Martinu. It was so special and one more example of how music is such a deep-seated and emotional need. I can't listen to Martinu now without thinking of her."

We love our music and it is a constant struggle to keep our two loves in balance.

"Ultimately for me, the priority has to be the patients," Dr. Kimberly said. "There have been a lot of times when I'd be in the middle of something at work and trying to tie up loose ends so I could get to rehearsal on time. I try to hurry, but then I think, 'It's not fair to the patient.' If you have a sick patient, you can't really pass them off to the next doctor. So I finish it up and have that last chat with the patient's family, even though I know I will be late. At least with the LSO, everyone will understand.

"When you're a doctor, the intensity of it comes home to you, literally. When I don't have rehearsal, sometimes I go home and lie in bed and think about my patients all night. And I wonder, 'Did I do the right thing? How are they feeling? How tragic that accident was . . .' I like to exercise a lot, but even as I'm running, I'm thinking about my patients. Even when I'm spending time with my kids, part of me is still thinking about my patients. It's a wheel that turns and turns constantly in your head. It's really hard to put aside.

"But when you're playing music, you can't have other thoughts in your mind. It's just the music. And you focus on that, and everything else goes away. In the end you can think back and put things in perspective a little bit.

"As exhausted as I sometimes am, especially if I've worked a 2 A.M. shift the night before, I drag myself to rehearsal. Why? Because I know that the minute I sit down and start playing, it's like a different switch goes on. It's a different focus. Everything about the day and whatever stress I had with the challenging patients just kind of disappears. I leave energetic and happy. That's why I'd drag myself to rehearsals. Because I know that at the end of it I will be so happy I did."

Scales to Scalpels is about the arts, compassion, and community as it is embodied by the musicians of the Longwood Symphony Orchestra and others. Somehow the scales we practiced so rigorously and passionately as children have led us from our musical instruments to other instruments, medical and surgical. Is this a new phenomenon? Or are the members of the Longwood Symphony Orchestra simply the modern-day practitioners of the age-old healing art of music?

2

A Pediatrician with a Violin

MY FATHER, DICK YIN WONG, was born in Honolulu in 1920. He grew up in poverty in a large Chinese immigrant family. Brilliant and determined, he graduated from the University of Hawaii as an accountant and took advantage of the GI Bill after World War II to further his education at Northwestern Law School in Chicago. My father was widely respected in his field of tax law and went on to become the nation's first Asian-American Federal District Court judge, appointed by President Gerald Ford.

During his time in Chicago, he developed an intense love of classical music and determined that his own children would have the gift of music instruction that he could not afford as a boy. Upon his return to Honolulu, my father met and married my mother, Lily Yee, an elementary school teacher who shared his passion for family, education, public service, and music. My four siblings and I were the lucky beneficiaries of their vision.

First Piano Lesson

One of my earliest childhood memories was that of our family's first piano lesson. Actually, it was my oldest sister's lesson, but it changed all our lives. Diane, at age seven, was deemed old enough to learn the piano, and a shiny new Story & Clark upright piano became the center of our home. In those days, we did not travel to a conservatory or piano studio. Rather, the itinerant piano teacher came to our house. The arrival of the piano, and the piano teacher, was a big event.

That first thirty-minute lesson passed quickly, with Diane and the teacher sharing the piano bench while I lay on the floor nearby, gazing at the patterns on the ceiling. She learned to put her thumbs on middle C and how each finger was numbered, one through five. She learned rudimentary scales and tackled the first few pages of John Thompson's *Modern Course for the Piano, Book I.* As soon as the teacher left and Diane went back to her dolls, I scrambled up onto the bench and played back everything I'd heard.

This went on for quite a while. Each week Diane would have her lesson, and each week I'd mimic what I'd heard, until finally my mother asked if I wanted to take piano lessons, too. I was three years old and ecstatic. In a sense, music has always been my primary language.

While I was the only one who started quite so young, all five of us were playing the piano by the age of seven. It wasn't until decades later that I learned how important this early training was for the neuroplasticity of our brains. At the time, it was simply what our family did. Once we demonstrated our aptitude and dedication to the piano, we were rewarded with the opportunity to choose a second instrument to study. My older sister, older brother, and I picked the violin and my younger sister fell in love with the cello. My baby brother, always the radical, tortured us with the trumpet.

There were many musical games at home. One of us would start a tune on the piano, and the others would have to create a way to embellish the melody. Or my sister would play a complex chord on the piano and I would have to listen from the other room and write down all of the notes. Liszt's "Hungarian Dance" became a hide-and-seek story about a wolf hunting in the forest, as we peeked out from behind the curtains. And Shostakovich's playful and ironic *Golden Age Polka* was arranged by my sister into a crazy four-hand duet. It served as a good-night ritual—hands crossing over each other's hands and music crescendo-ing until we ended, triple *forte,* in peals of laughter.

As we got older, my sister Diane, the organizer, started transcribing viola parts into third violin parts, so that the family (without the renegade brass player) could play string quartets. We played at our school, at church, family Christmas parties, and for my elderly grandparents. When the Hawaii Youth Symphony created a Junior Orchestra, we all joined eagerly. At concerts, the conductor would introduce the ensemble and explain that HJO was an orchestra for children aged twelve to fifteen. I was taught to stand up from my stand in the back of the violin section and stamp my foot indignantly ". . . *and* one ten-year-old," he would clarify, with a smile.

Each year, the Junior Orchestra toured Hawaii's outer islands. We'd wake up at five in the morning to take the twenty-minute flight from Honolulu to perform for the school children living on Maui, Kauai, Molokai, and even the sparsely populated Lanai, which at the time only had a single schoolhouse. Many of the children in rural Hawaii, most of whom were our age, had had no exposure to classical music in their schools. We took delight in sitting with them in the lunchyard, demonstrating our instruments.

GIVING BACK TO OHANA

I was fortunate to attend Punahou School, one of the country's oldest independent schools. Originally founded in 1841 by missionaries to educate their own children, it is now a racial and cultural melting pot of students from the Hawaiian Islands. Punahou celebrates diversity and creativity and has centered its curriculum on academic excellence, the arts, and community service. The school proudly counts among its alumni Juilliard musicians, Tony-nominated actors, entrepreneurs such as AOL founder Steve Case, and statesmen, including—President Barack Obama. Having been blessed with many gifts, the students are all encouraged to give back to our *ohana*—our larger family—the community.

I started volunteering weekly at the Shriners Hospital for Crippled Children when I turned fifteen. The children there were mainly from the Polynesian Islands, where *talipes equinovaris*, or "clubfoot," was a common birth defect. They would be brought to Honolulu for orthopedic correction, spend weeks in recuperation and therapy, then return to their homes in Polynesia. Because many required multiple procedures over a number of years, Shriners Hospital became a second home to them. While I did not understand the surgical details, I soon learned the rhythm of their stays and became close to many of the patients.

I became interested in how homesickness and under-stimulation could make their pain worse and slow their recovery. I worked with the staff to think of ways to alleviate their physical and emotional pain. We didn't spend a lot of time watching television at the hospital, and DVDs and videos did not exist yet. Sometimes we'd bring books to read and games to play. Sometimes we would watch *Sesame Street*. But there would always be music. I'd taught myself the guitar by then, and so the afternoons would pass singing or trying to teach them the guitar and piano. I even brought my high school string quartet to visit them. The music would make them smile—for a brief afternoon, the pain, homesickness, and monotony of the hospital would fade away.

My experience at Shriners Hospital was transformative for me. By the time I left the Islands for Harvard, I had decided that my career would be devoted to children and somehow incorporate music, health, community service, and education. But I had no idea which would take precedence. Would I be a musician? A teacher? A music therapist? A doctor?

My freshman Expository Writing advisor understood my dilemma far better than I did. Each week's assignment sent me to look at my options from a different perspective. One week was an observation piece in the busy lobby of the Mt. Auburn Hospital. Another was to write a reflection about teaching in the second grade class of Buckingham Browne and Nichols School. Still another was a review of a classical music concert.

By this time, I'd met some of the other residents in my dormitory, including a young cellist named Yo-Yo Ma, a dashing violinist named Lynn Chang (my future husband), and a brilliant multitalented pianist named Richard Kogan. Even as undergraduates, these three were already making a huge impact on the international music scene. The reality of being a small musical Hawaiian fish in a big New England pond began to sink in. While this certainly tempered my dreams for a musical career, my musical knowledge and love for the art form flourished as I became one of the luckiest groupies on campus.

During those heady years during the mid-1970s, my friends and I became members of a pickup orchestra organized by a music graduate student; whenever Yo-Yo, Lynn, or Richard wanted to try out a new concerto, we were there. Rehearsals were in the evening, while the concerts, always sold out, often went on until midnight. I even found myself in the unlikely situation of playing piano for a cellist friend (who later became a radiologist) for a cello master class led by Rostropovich.

MY FATHER'S WISDOM

At Christmas break of my senior year in college, all five children in my family were home to celebrate the holidays together. By then, my older sister had returned to Hawaii to begin her law career. The three middle ones were in college on the Mainland and the youngest, Steven, was still a high school junior.

On the day after Christmas, we were waiting for my father to come home from work to celebrate my younger sister's birthday. At about 6:30 P.M. a call came from the hospital for my mother. "It's about your husband. It's urgent. Can you come down to the hospital now? Is there someone who can come with you?" Older brother David prepared to drive my mother on the ten-minute trip. I was assigned to cancel dinner reservations.

After that . . . no word for hours.

Finally, David and Mom returned home, along with my father's best friend. "Dad's passed away. He had a heart attack at the Y after running. He collapsed in the stairwell and never regained consciousness."

"What!? Why didn't you call us from the hospital? Couldn't we have come down to say good-bye? How could this happen?" He was only fifty-eight years old.

The days that followed were a blur. I remember having a long talk with Reverend Grant Lee, my close friend and pastor. I asked him why God would do this. I asked him what God meant by leaving our family alone. At the time I remember being angry by Grant's inability to explain the unexplainable. No, He was not angry with us. Yes, all things happen for a reason. But sometimes it is not clear at the time. I think I told him that was not acceptable. I recall he just looked at me with compassion and no words.

After the funeral, we had to decide what to do next. Diane and Steve were home, so Mom was not left alone. The other three of us were in the middle of our academic year. What would Dad have wanted us to do? Of course, we knew the answer. It was to go back to the Mainland, and to honor his memory by doing as well as he would have expected of us. So I returned, heavy-hearted, to Harvard, where I was now majoring in East Asian Studies. I took my final pre-med exams and completed a forty-two-page analysis of the Schumann

Piano Quintet. The professor gave me an A-minus because it was late.

It was not until I was much older that I came to terms with my father's death and I understood his wisdom and foresight. He had given us the gift of music. He had taught us to be intellectually curious and fiercely independent. And when he died, we learned that, despite his modest salary as a federal judge, he had had the foresight to set up educational trusts for all five of his children. Thanks to his vision, even after his death, we were all able to attend college and graduate school with very few loans, and my mother was secure for the rest of her life.

HARMONY OUT OF DISCORD

That spring, I was accepted to NYU Medical School and graduated *magna cum laude* from Harvard. My mother, still grieving, could not bring herself to travel to Boston for my graduation.

I chose New York because I felt the need to explore another new city. I went there to pursue medicine, but discovered a richness in the arts that I'd never before experienced. Thanks to our Student Activities Office, tickets to the ballet (Baryshnikov had just taken the helm at the American Ballet Theater), Metropolitan Opera, and New York Philharmonic were all only five dollars! And Broadway shows were free the week before they were reviewed. I was on cloud nine.

I realized I was not a typical medical student. In fact, in some ways, I was unprepared for the academic rigors of medical school. Many of my classmates were biochemistry majors—I was a social scientist with some knowledge about the Chinese revolution and a passion for Brahms. I started out trying to emulate these brilliant classmates—studying for six hours a day, burying myself in the library and trying to memorize my anatomy textbook. It was rough going. My favorite was the anatomy coloring book, which is not as infantile as it sounds. But it kept my hands busy while I memorized all those Latin names.

In the social sciences, I could just flip to the back of the chapter, read the author's conclusion, and work my way forward from the beginning again to pick up pertinent facts. It was a rude shock after the first exams to find that one can't learn body parts that way. Somewhere along the line, one misses a few key nerves, veins, and arteries.

To occupy myself, I started exploring the NYU medical building. The dormitory is attached through hallways to all of the classrooms and labs. One evening, to my delight, I discovered a baby grand piano on the top floor of the rehab hospital. This became my refuge at night when I needed stretch my fingers over Bach to let medical facts settle in my brain.

As my fellow classmates got to know each other better, we realized that NYU had chosen a medical school class full of artists. One friend had been a professional recorder player. A few were fine pianists. One had directed summer stock theatre in upstate New York, and another did lighting for the drama department at University of Massachusetts at Amherst. We found other actors and singers in the class—and by the second semester, our first year medical school class put on NYU's first full-length musical, *You're a Good Man, Charlie Brown* in a transformed lecture hall. The money we raised from our three performances was matched by the dean's office. With it, we were able to buy a new upright piano for the student lounge.

After that, the NYU Chamber Music Society was launched—
we put on a series of concerts including Bach's Brandenburg
Concerto No. 4 with full orchestra and my classmate as one
of the recorder soloists.

As soon as I added my music, theater, and art back into
the mix, my grades went up. And as soon as we started to get
out of the classrooms into clinical rotations, all the studying
suddenly made sense. If I saw a case, then went back to study
the pathophysiology, the medical details that were so difficult
to memorize out of context clicked when I could appreciate
their relevance for the patient. It was not unlike learning a
complex new piece. I could practice the individual phrases;
but until the notes lined up right and the tune was discern-
ible, it was not music.

There is a quote I love from Plutarch, circa 180 A.D., that
I discovered in my wanderings through the NYU library at
this time:

"Medicine, to produce health, must examine disease" and
"Music, to create harmony, must investigate discord."

MOVING FORWARD

In October of my fourth medical school year, I married my
college sweetheart Lynn Chang, now a professional violinist
whose parents were both doctors. Since he was teaching in
Cambridge, I moved back to Boston after the wedding and
arranged for most of my fourth-year rotations to be in Boston-
area hospitals.

In his autobiography, *The Edge of the Primeval Forest*,
Dr. Albert Schweitzer refers to "the fellowship of those who
bear the mark of pain,"[1] asserting that "Those who have

learnt by experience what physical pain and bodily anguish mean, belong together all the world over; they are united by a secret bond." My father's death left me with a question that I still ponder often—is it harder to lose a loved one suddenly without warning, or slowly, after a long battle that can drain a family mentally and financially? There is no good answer to this, nor is there any right answer. Each brings its own pain and requires its own healing.

Sadly, Dad was not there for the big events of my life—my graduations, marriage, and birth of my two children—but I have also reasoned that my father, the impatient perfectionist with an insatiable curiosity and love of learning, who did not like to lose at anything—chess, basketball, Name-That-Classical-Tune—would have been a lousy chronic patient. Death on his own terms, sudden and quick, was likely the best thing for him. It was not necessarily the best thing for those he left behind. But then, there isn't really a "best way" to do it, is there?

But it is in his honor and memory that we as a family have learned to move forward. I have often been able to use this knowledge, as a member of "the fellowship of those who bear the mark of pain," with my own pediatric patients. Over the years, I have cared for several children whose journey has included losing one or both parents. Some need close care right after the loss. Others react much later—sometimes years later. It is at these times that I feel fortunate to be able to be their doctor for the long term, and to be able to say, with all sincerity, "I know what you are going through."

3

Music and Healers, from Apollo to Dr. Albert Schweitzer

"MUSIC IS A KIND OF MEDICINE," says Dr. Tom Sheldon, a wiry man whose wise eyes reveal a twinkle of humor. Tom is a radiation oncologist who serves as Medical Director of Radiation Oncology at Concord Hospital in New Hampshire. Each week, he drives down to Boston through daunting traffic to play oboe with us. Longwood Avenue is a second home to him—Dr. Sheldon did his medical school and residency here in Boston, finishing in 1984. He has been a cancer doctor ever since.

"I am often dealing with life-threatening situations," he said. "I have to do the smartest thing possible and do it in a way that is as humane as possible. It is a big challenge and a constant struggle.

"And it's not something that is easy to share. It's not like at the end of the day, we docs sit around and say, 'I had the most depressing case today.' We talk about the intellectually or technically challenging cases, but we don't share the emotional side. It's just not done! You go through years and years and years of this with few ways to lighten this load.

"But suddenly in my life, there was music again. I find it very healing. I can express myself in a way that frees me of a lot of that emotional weight that was added from years of oncology practice. I can't explain how it works, and I don't really understand why it works so well. But it's real."

There is the old Biblical proverb: "Physician, heal thyself" (Luke: 4:23). That is still good advice, and music can make it happen.

As medicine for patients, a dose of music is easy and often free. "Music is so ubiquitous. It is everywhere. It is definitely the number one art form that we all take in. Just turn on the radio. Music is always on."

A WAITING-ROOM MAGAZINE CHANGED HIS LIFE

Dr. Sheldon played oboe as a young man but focused on it far less while he was building his medical career. In the early 2000s he nearly threw away his musical future, quite literally. He was in the process of tossing out old waiting room magazines (yes, it happens!) when his eye happened to land on an article about doctors' orchestras, which inspired him to give our group a try.

Dr. Sheldon was already a recognized expert in the field of radiation oncology. But joining the LSO put him back at the bottom of the ladder again. "I'm considered to be well respected in my field," he said. "Here I am, a respected senior physician, and I start playing in a high-quality orchestra on a difficult instrument after a twenty-year hiatus. Rehearsals, much less performances, were intimidating and stressful: in a word, intense. It was also an intense time to be in the LSO. Jonathan [McPhee] was applying pressure, trying to raise the bar and get us to play up to our potential. I used to get very nervous before every rehearsal. The oboe is a solo instrument, only two playing. You can't hide like a player in the middle of the violin section. A conductor the caliber of Jonathan hears everything you do. My intonation was inconsistent (mostly sharp). My music reading skills were sad. Luckily, I have always been blessed with good rhythm, and that seemed to hold up. The biggest problem I would describe as auditory confusion. There is a lot to listen to and follow in orchestra playing, and I just could not separate it out. So much of it was confusing noise. It has taken years of work to get chill at rehearsals and finally to get chill at concerts. But I worked my way up to it. I can play, I can hear, and I can understand. It's great. I really enjoy it."

Many of his fellow LSO musicians have a similar story to tell. Nearly all gave up or severely curtailed music during the early years of medical training, only to discover what a big hole that left in their lives.

"I have enormously deep and profound experiences dealing with patients and their families in crisis every day," Sheldon went on, "and it is expressed in my music. Even if music does take some time out of the medicine, I believe it works as an advantage to my patients. I think I am a smarter and more sensitive doctor because I play music. I think more clearly and am emotionally more available to my patients. In the end it's not an issue of balancing music and medicine. They became one thing. The medicine makes me a better musician, and the music makes me a better doctor."

This human element to medicine comes up time and time again. There are few things nowadays that machines can't do nearly as well as craftspersons. No computer algorithm can replace a well-reasoned history and physical. No lab result is helpful without medical context and a physician's interpretation. So many things need that human touch. Take cutting a reed for the mouthpiece of an oboe. If you ever pressed a blade of grass between your thumbs and blew to make a blatting sound, you have a general idea how an oboe works, though an oboe uses two blades, called reeds, vibrating against one another, which results in a sound that is mellow, sometimes mournful, and often profound. Trumpets are played by buzzing the lips into a metal mouthpiece. Saxophones are played by blowing through a thick flat slice of bamboo called a reed. But oboists use a much more delicate double reed, and one that consists of two tapered bits of bamboo cane that meet at a flat point less than a quarter inch wide.

There are machines that purport to make these reeds and you can buy them at music stores. But most serious oboists know: you have to manufacture them yourself. Ask Dr. Sheldon: "Everybody's mouth is different. Everybody's lips have a different embouchure [the way they purse their lips to play]. So that means you have to learn how to create them to suit your unique requirements. It is a very complex process that starts with a tube of bamboo and a metal tube!"

He carries in his pocket a small metal case, slightly longer and thicker than a cigarette case. He flips it open. Nestled close together inside are about a dozen objects that look like custom-tied fishing lures, but without the showy colorful wings and attention-getting flaps used by fly fishers. Instead, the end of each has two fine-grained reeds pressed together like elongated hands held in prayer.

"They say you have to make a bushel basket of them before you really get it right. And you need more than one because they respond differently, depending whether it's humid out or cold. They also change slightly as you use them. They require a breaking-in period, and then they degrade after a while. A good reed might last for five or six hours. Occasionally you will get a reed that you can play on occasionally for six weeks and it's great each time. You need to be able to scrape the reed and make adjustments on the spot. At any one time I might have ten reeds that are in different stages of adjustment. I'm getting much better at it. I can get a playable reed in about twenty minutes." "You can see how narrow and how fine the tip is," Dr. Sheldon said proudly. "The hardest thing about playing the oboe is making these reeds. It can take half of your practice time. You start with a piece of bamboo that is folded in half, and then you. . . ." He demonstrates, looking like a surgeon using a scalpel to make incremental whittles on a tiny stick. Which is sort of what he is.

Even under the best of conditions, the sound balance of each reed is slightly different. "There is a difference in how easy you can speak a note, how loud they are, and whether the pitch is a little high or a little low You could pull out three reeds and the pitch relationship between my B and my A would be a little different on each one of those reeds."

On top of all that, Dr. Sheldon said you even need different reeds for different pieces of music. "You might need a very hard, raucous reed to play some of Mahler. I need a very different kind of reed when I play Vivaldi: very flexible and a little more Baroque-sounding."

But Dr. Sheldon said that Maestro McPhee, whose main instrument was also oboe, taught him the most important lesson as an oboist, which can translate to the practice of medicine as well. "For a long time I was struggling with reed-making. Jonathan took me aside and said, 'Remember: in the end, your sound is *here*,' and he put his two index fingers to his head. Your sound first and foremost is in your mind. And it's true. Two oboists could play the same piece of music with the same reed on the same instrument and they would sound completely different."

Dr. Sheldon said that kind of ultra-customization serves him well as a doctor. The parable of the reeds has taught him that no two patients are ever the same. And as with the reed, it is what is in your head as well as your heart that gets the best result.

APOLLO'S CHILDREN

Musician-physicians like Dr. Sheldon have been getting a lot of press recently, but the phenomenon has existed almost as long as there have been doctors. Perhaps modern doctors haven't wanted to be associated with anything as seemingly frivolous as music. But my informal surveys at conferences I've attended through the years have shown that seventy to eighty percent of physicians have had musical training as children. So it's been a semi-secret passion for them. But it was not always that way. Here is a timeline of musician-physicians in history.

Music in Ancient Times

Music has been a part of medicine since its earliest days. Rhythmic chanting and dancing were used for healing in pre-scientific societies around the world, and are still practiced among many cultures, notably Native American in all their variety throughout the Western Hemisphere. The Greek god, Apollo, served triple duty, as god of the sun, healing, and music. His son, Aesculapius, is the God of Medicine.

But there is also something of a tradition of using music even in science-based treatment. Hippocrates, the fourth-century B.C. physician we know as the "Father of Western Medicine" and author/namesake of the Hippocratic Oath, also believed that music, as well as poetry and literature, were an integral part of medicine.[1]

The Middle Ages

Many of Hippocrates' successors agreed. During the Middle Ages, when the cutting edge of intellectual development shifted to the Muslim world, two seminal figures supported music as a tool of medicine, if not actually a branch of medicine. Turco-Persian Al-Farabi (known in the West as Alpharabius) considered music as therapy in his treatise *Meaning of the Intellect* (circa A.D. 925) and in his massive twenty-one-volume *Kitab al-musiqa al-kabir* (*Great Book on Music*).[2] He compared music and medicine, saying that each drew its "principles from natural science, and is learned principally from sensory experience acquired through anatomy."[3]

The Central Asian Ibn Sina's (known in the West as Avicenna) encyclopedic 11th-century *Kitab al-Shifa'* (*The Book of Healing*) included a chapter on what today would be termed "music therapy."[4] He analyzed many different musical intervals and asserted that music's ability to "delight the soul" could have a positive effect on mental and physical health.[5]

THE NINETEENTH CENTURY

Russian composer Alexander Borodin (1883–1887) considered himself only a "Sunday musician." The relatively small size of his body of work, which includes his beloved Polovtsian Dances (made popular in the musical *Kismet* as "Stranger in Paradise"), can be blamed on the demands of his primary career, teaching chemistry at the St. Petersburg Academy of Medicine in Russia, where he was one of the first researchers to link cholesterol with heart disease.[6] The medical world remembers him for founding the School of Medicine for Women in St. Petersburg. The musical world remembers him as part of a circle of nationalistic Russian composers of his day called "The Five," including Mussorgsky and Rimsky-Korsakov.[7]

Borodin, according to "Blue" Gene Tyranny in the *All Music Guide,* "wrote music of great originality and beauty— bold orchestral tone poems on exotic lands and subjects, as well as Russian nationalist works influenced by folk melodies and featuring astonishing harmonic and rhythmic innovation (chords in fourths, harmonies with non-harmonic 'added tones,' quasi-jazz syncopation)."[8]

In France, Dr. René Laennec (1781–1826), an accomplished flutist, applied his knowledge of the sound transmission through wooden flutes to invent the now ubiquitous and indispensible stethoscope, which he named from the Greek words *stethos* (meaning chest) and *skopos* (observer). Previously, doctors would press their ears directly to the chests of their patients to listen to their heartbeats—a practice that offended the sensibilities of some of the more proper ladies.

Laennec might have had a French medical colleague in Hector Berlioz (1803–1869) had it not been for the composer's suffering a traumatic experience in medical school that caused him to abandon the profession. Aspiring doctors were required to acquire their own cadavers for dissection class. "At that terrible charnel-house," he wrote in his *Memoirs*, "fragments of ribs, the grinning heads and gaping skulls, the bloody quagmire underfoot and the atrocious smell it gave off, the swarms of sparrows wrangling over scraps of lung, the rats in the corner gnawing the bleeding vertebrae—such a feeling of revulsion possessed me that I leapt through the window of the dissecting room and fled for home as though death and all his hideous train were at my heels." [9]

He turned that force of feeling and of observation into a repertoire of great orchestral pieces: one can almost picture the horrors of cadaver-hunting in his *Symphonie fantastique* and *Grande messe des morts* (*Great Mass of the Dead*).

BRAHMS AND BILLROTH

As music and medicine advanced in the nineteenth century, so did the links between them. For example, composer Johannes Brahms and Dr. Christian Albert Theodor Billroth developed a rich and unusual collaboration. Master musician Brahms was fascinated by medicine. Innovative surgeon Billroth loved music. He was a talented amateur classical violinist and pianist who, besides his many medical articles, wrote a famous treatise proposing a scientific approach to the appreciation of music.

The two men formed a close friendship during their fertile years in Austria in the late 1800s.

Raised by his grandparents, who were both opera singers, Billroth proved to be a passionate devotee of music, but an indifferent medical student. Nevertheless, once he went into practice, he became far more passionate about medicine and medical research. Billroth is widely regarded as the father of abdominal surgery, and is credited with the development of the first successful procedures to treat cancers of the esophagus, stomach, and colon. Two hemigastrectomy procedures—surgical techniques that reroute the intestine—bear his name (Billroth I and Billroth II) and are still used in surgery today.[10] In addition, he promoted the advancement of the institution of surgical residencies and the profession of nursing.

You wouldn't think Billroth would have had time for music, but he devoted many evenings to playing in musical salons with his friend Johannes Brahms, who trusted Billroth's advice and let him have first look, and first listen, to many of his pieces composed during this time. Brahms dedicated his two Opus 51 string quartets to this musical doctor who also attended many orchestra rehearsals and occasionally took up the baton himself.

Billroth was touched by the dedications, yet wrote to a colleague, "I am afraid these dedications will keep our names in memory longer than the best work we have done; for us, not very complimentary, but beautiful for humanity, which, with the right instinct, considers art more immortal than science. It is a human fact that love weighs more than great respect."[11]

A heavy smoker, Billroth died of lung disease in 1894 at age sixty-five. He left behind an essay, "Wer ist musikalisch?"

("What does it mean to be musical?"), published posthumously. Like so much of his medical work, he was ahead of his time. The treatise offers prescient insights about how the human mind perceives and processes music. He wrote in a letter, "It is one of the superficialities of our time to see in science and in art two opposites; imagination is the mother of both." [12]

THE TWENTIETH CENTURY

The twentieth century found still other musicians and composers who started their lives in the healing arts. Stormy serialist composer and conductor Giuseppe Sinopoli earned his doctorate, not in music, but medicine from Padua University, writing his thesis on criminal anthropology and later taking up archaeology. [13] Pianist and composer Samuel Zyman graduated from medical school in Mexico before leaving for New York to attend the Juilliard School. Zyman never looked back: he is now a professor of music theory and composition at that famed New York conservatory. Still, Zyman finds that he uses medical metaphors to get his point across to young composers from time to time: he has compared the energy that surges through the climax of the Sacrificial Dance in Stravinsky's *Rite of Spring* to the electrophysiology of the heart.

For Dr. Rupa Marya, a San Francisco-born physician of Indian descent, music and medicine have always had a delicate balance. Dr. Marya spends six months practicing medicine and six months recording and performing as lead singer in her band, Rupa and the April Fishes. In a 2008 interview on NPR, she explained, "after my first year of internship, I went to my program director and said, 'Listen, I'll be a terrible doctor if I'm not an artist, and I'll be a terrible artist if I'm not a doctor." Marya goes on to observe that on occasion her patients are the musical inspiration for her songs.[14]

Former New York Philharmonic conductor emeritus Zubin Mehta studied medicine at the college level in his native India before moving abroad and switching to classical music studies. Sir Jeffrey Tate, too, completed his medical studies prior to devoting his life to music, becoming one of the most celebrated opera conductors of our time. And there's Eddie Henderson, the jazz trumpeter who put himself through Howard University medical school by playing gigs, but then returned to music after ten years and has since played with Herbie Hancock, Art Blakey, Dexter Gordon, McCoy Tyner, and others. He did his residency in psychiatry, but was a general practitioner from 1975 to 1986.[15]

CONTINUING THE TRADITION

Orchestras like the Longwood Symphony Orchestra are made up of medical professionals who, unlike the composers and musicians mentioned in the previous section, strive to balance their music with their medicine. In the United States, there is the seventy-member Los Angeles Doctors Symphony Orchestra that was founded in 1953; the Doctors Orchestral Society of New York was founded in 1938; there is also the Texas Medical Center Orchestra, the Life Sciences Orchestra in Michigan, the Doctors Orchestra of Houston, and the Philadelphia Doctors Chamber Orchestra, all of which have formed in the past half century. The phenomenon is international as well, with the Australian Doctors Orchestra, the London-based European Doctors Orchestra, the Bucharest (Romania) Physicians Orchestra, and the Berlin-based World Doctor's Orchestra, among many others, all thriving. Though nearly all were founded independently, they follow remarkably similar precepts and tap into an identical yearning among musician-physicians to continue their music. Although they do not share the same philanthropic model as the Longwood Symphony, many donate proceeds from their concerts to medical causes.

THE ULTIMATE MUSICIAN-PHYSICIAN

The individual I consider the greatest of all musician-physicians is Nobel-Peace Prize laureate Dr. Albert Schweitzer. A musician, philosopher, humanitarian, and physician, Dr. Schweitzer offers inspiration to all of us in the Longwood Symphony Orchestra.

Dr. Schweitzer's life has been the subject of at least six published biographies, countless magazine and newspaper articles, and at least three films including the widely seen 1957 film *Albert Schweitzer* starring Phillip Eckert, and a 1990 TV movie, *Schweitzer,* starring Malcolm McDowell.

Dr. Schweitzer was born in 1875 in Alsace (then part of Germany) into a family of pastors and organists. Like his family before him, he, too, became a pastor and theologian and continued to play piano and organ professionally into the 1950s. Schweitzer received his Ph.D. in philosophy in 1855 and published a biography of Johann Sebastian Bach in 1905, quickly followed by his best-seller *The Quest of the Historical Jesus,* published in 1906. At the age of thirty, upon learning of the primitive state of medical care in sub-Saharan Africa, he turned his back on a comfortable life as theologian, writer, and musician, and went to medical school. Later, Schweitzer wrote, "I decided to make life my agreement."[16]

In 1913, Schweitzer and his wife were assigned to the village of Lambaréné in what was then called French Equatorial Africa (today the nation of Gabon). Traveling up the Ogooué River into the primeval rainforest, Dr. Schweitzer underwent a spiritual awakening about the sanctity of life. His flash of insight was summarized as "Reverence for Life," and it became his life's watchword.

Lucky, lucky Lambaréné! When Schweitzer arrived there he found a place with all the disadvantages of poverty, but with a rich spiritual life. He founded a hospital, soon to be world-famous, where he researched and did battle with the many tropical afflictions of the people there. He also built a church, where he served as pastor and sometime organist. Dr. Schweitzer devoted the rest of his life (except for a time late in World War I when he was imprisoned by the French as an enemy national) to the practice of Reverence for Life, through caring for the Gabonese, preaching, and music, all with the aim of improving the well-being of the Gabonese.

He was awarded the Nobel Prize for Peace in 1952. In Schweitzer-spirited fashion, he used the $33,000 in prize money to build a special treatment center for leprosy (then called Hansen's Disease) in his beloved Lambaréné. He died in 1965 and his gravesite in Lambaréné still attracts pilgrims.[17, 18, 19, 20] More importantly, his hospital is still vibrant and growing under the leadership of Schweitzer-spirited physician Dr. Lachlan Forrow, and will celebrate its centenary in 20, hopefully with the music provided by members of the LSO.

His life and work have profoundly inspired not just me, but nearly all the musician-physicians of the Longwood Symphony Orchestra. One might say he is our patron saint.

4

The Longwood Symphony Orchestra Finds Its Own Lambaréné

BOSTON IS BLESSED WITH MANY classical music organizations large, medium, and small, from the world-class Boston Symphony and the widely-known Boston Pops, to community orchestras like the New Philharmonia Orchestra and Civic Symphony in my own town. When I returned to Massachusetts for my pediatric residency at Mass. General Hospital shortly after getting married, I joined the Longy Chamber Orchestra at the Longy School in Cambridge. This small community ensemble consisted of amateurs and professionals who performed music of the classical era. The group was led by Endel Kalam, a violist and long-time member of the Boston Symphony Orchestra, whose warmth and passion for the music was infectious. Because my daughter was born in July 1985, just as I was starting my final year of residency at

41

Massachusetts General Hospital, I did not play in the fateful summer concert, at which Endel Kalam quietly collapsed and died onstage of a heart attack after conducting the final bars of the slow movement of a Haydn Symphony. We were devastated by the loss of this beloved man and the sense of community he had engendered in this intimate community orchestra, comforted only in knowing that he died while doing what he loved most.

At that point, the Longy began to go through a transition. Kalam's successors thought that they would change the model of the orchestra into more of a teaching orchestra for the students than a community/school ensemble. A number of Longy musicians including me began looking for a place where we could feel as comfortable as we had with Maestro Kalam. It turns out, there was one that had formed just across town.

"I Bet You're Right"

Sometime in late 1983 or early 1984, two chaplains at New England Deaconess Hospital (now a part of the Beth Israel Deaconess Medical Center of Boston) in the Longwood medical area had what turned out to be a fateful conversation.

They were Rev. Dr. Guy Steele, Sr. Director of Pastoral Care, and the Rev. Charles W. Kessler, a United Methodist Minister on the staff. Their jobs were to tend to the spiritual needs of patients and family members as they face some of the most difficult moments of their lives. It's hard to imagine two more comforting figures, the slender Rev. Steele with his friendly Midwestern accent, and the warm-voiced Rev. Kessler whose searching eyes express his compassion. Both are also musicians—Rev. Steele a trumpet player and Rev. Kessler a violinist. Both played in small informal chamber groups and were struck by how many of the musicians they played with were health professionals.

Rev. Kessler said "I can give you the exact words Rev. Steele said, when I spoke with him for this book. 'Charlie, don't you suppose with all the physicians and other people who play music in the medical world that there is a symphony orchestra walking into this medical area every day?'"

Rev. Kessler added, "I said something like, 'I bet you're right.'"

These simple words might have floated away as just another conversation. How many conversations like that have all of us had? But these were men of action as well as men of the cloth and music. So they started asking around, contacting their friends who were musicians, and asking if they would like to do more formally what they'd already been doing for a long time: getting together to play as physician musicians.

Although to my knowledge a survey has not yet been done, the general consensus is that about seventy-five percent of people in the medical and science community had at least a year of instrumental music training as children. The attention to detail, neurologic coordination, and element of disciplined creativity required of a young musician helped many of us become who we are today.

It took only a few months for Steele and Kessler to organize their "medical orchestra." Key aid came from Rev. Steele's wife, Nalora, an opera singer, music teacher, and choral conductor, who was organizing a community choir she had named the Longwood Chorus, after the Longwood Medical Area where she did her recruiting.

In the fall of 1984, Steele and Kessler gathered nine musicians (including themselves) and scheduled the debut of the ensemble they dubbed the Longwood Chamber Orchestra. "We wanted to do something fun," said Rev. Steele, and they settled on Haydn's "Toy Symphony," which was performed, with the customary addition of various whistles, toy instruments, and other sound effects, under the baton of Mrs. Steele at St. Paul's Church in Boston just before Christmas 1984.

Thus our orchestra had its own symbolic nativity that year. And the baby seemed healthy, albeit tiny. Other musicians along Longwood Avenue began to inquire and Steele and Kessler decided that if they were really serious about organizing a full-scale Longwood Symphony Orchestra, they'd need an experienced conductor. One of the early members proposed a young wunderkind graduate student out of the New England Conservatory, Aaron Kula, who shared the founders' ambition to build a real orchestra.

Kula helped arrange the group's first full-scale engagement, celebrating the rededication of the Stoneham Library in Stoneham, Massachusetts, about ten miles north of Boston. Noting that the date, March 21, 1985, coincided with the three hundredth anniversary of Bach's birth, Kula, Steele and Kessler programmed an ambitious all-Bach concert of "Jesu, Joy of Man's Desiring," the "Air" from the Orchestral Suite in D major, and the second, third, and fourth Brandenburg Concertos.

The concert was a great success, and the nascent LSO was asked to play the Brandenburgs again at New England

Deaconess Hospital at few weeks later. These successes produced positive word-of-mouth for the LSO. But the real surge in membership occurred over the ensuing weeks after word got around that Maestro Kula had landed the LSO an enviable booking at the Hatch Shell on the Boston Esplanade overlooking the Charles River, which you may recognize as the spot where the Boston Pops plays its televised concerts each Fourth of July. We've continued the tradition of playing an annual summer concert on the Esplanade ever since.

The Right Man at the Time

Among the people attracted to join the LSO were me and my friends from the Longy Orchestra. I heard about the LSO from Dr. Len Zon, a trumpet player and resident at the Deaconess Hospital who was one of the LSO's original members. In keeping with its informal roots, the LSO at the time had no audition process; anyone who wanted to play could get in. We've come a long way since then: we have instituted formal auditions, and performance standards have risen to the point where I'm not even sure I myself would be admitted if I auditioned now.

But Maestro Kula was the right man for the job at that time. Clarinetist Mark Gebhardt recalls: "Aaron was okay to get us started. I don't think it's easy to conduct this group. For a non-physician to conduct a group of people who are used to calling the shots all day, and who are distracted when they come in, *and* then to get this group to focus and to give up control—all of that is not easy for any conductor. In rehearsal there's an expectation of a certain amount of musician preparedness for the rehearsal, and that almost never happened.

And that gets frustrating. Kula tolerated that fairly well. And we played some *great* pieces."

Kula helped the LSO elbow its way into the Boston musical world. We tackled some very ambitious programs in those years and cemented our reputation as something beyond a "hobby" organization.

When the season began in September 1985, the orchestra had grown to a sizable seventy-five members. Back then, the rehearsals were held at the New England Deaconess Hospital's cafeteria and after several moves wound up in the band room of Boston Latin School.

It felt like home to me. From the beginning, there was something special about the musicians of the LSO. Busy professionals, many with families, who were doing meaningful and sometimes heartbreaking work during the day, all found something in the camaraderie and musical experience that made them want to carve out time from their personal lives to give to the orchestra. It seemed to fill a deep inner need. Word spread in the medical community. In just a few short years, the LSO would grow into a full symphonic orchestra of nearly a hundred musicians, and a nearly equal number of alternates.

Jordan Hall

One of the first and best (and most expensive) decisions made by our founders was to perform at New England Conservatory's Jordan Hall in Boston. This gem of a performance space, located a block down Huntington Avenue from the legendary Symphony Hall in the Back Bay area, was built between 1901 and 1903 as part of the New England Conservatory. It's named for NEC trustee and benefactor Eben D. Jordan II, a scion of the Jordan Marsh department store family. It is now listed on the National Registry of Historic Places. I'm proud to say that Jordan Hall is universally recognized as having some of the most flawlessly crystalline acoustics of any hall in America, if not the world.

The exterior of Jordan Hall gives little hint of the magnificent interior. It is a dignified but unremarkable squarish three-story concrete building in the Georgian style. You enter on the Gainsborough Street side up a short flight of steps between two light poles, each with four white globes. The poles are decorated with a motif of lyres, which continues inside.

Once inside, dark brown leatherette seats and dark green carpeting set off the light wood wall panels on the walls and ceiling. The center of attention is a majestic pipe organ that fills the entire back wall of the stage. Jordan Hall seems to have been built like an old-time sailing ship—one of those elegant Spanish caravels perhaps, all curved wood with few flat, horizontal surfaces other than the stage itself. The sharply raked orchestra section affords good views to all; the horseshoe-shaped balcony embraces the audience and draws it close to the performers. And our "groupies" love it, too. At an intimate 1019 seats (versus 2625 for Symphony Hall), our audiences are practically in our laps, an experience of musical intimacy that cannot be realized in the much larger Boston Symphony Hall (2,625 seats) down the street.

Then there are the legendary acoustics. The shape of the theatre, its materials, and even its decorations help to distribute the sound as well as any electronic mixing board.

Sitting in the back of the balcony you can hear a whispered conversation between orchestra members on stage—even while the orchestra is playing! Think of Jordan Hall as a giant musical instrument: a huge horn with the stage as its mouthpiece and the auditorium as its grand bell.

Aspiring to perform in Jordan Hall was an act of hubris on the part of Rev. Kessler, Maestro Kula, and the Steeles. That toddler form of the LSO was hardly up to Jordan Hall's musical standards in terms of quality. But there's nothing wrong with having high hopes. One of our biggest challenges each year is to raise the money for the rental of this venerable space. But it's been well worth it. I can't overstate how much Jordan Hall itself has spurred the LSO. Playing in that hallowed space inspired us all to push ourselves to play better in order to be worthy of it, and it still does. We love it for that reason. The better we have played over the years, the prouder we have felt.

Rehearsals back at the Boston Latin School give us only a vague sense of what our performance will actually sound like in Jordan Hall. The band room there flattens and distorts our sound. The brass can't hear the strings and the cellos strain to hear the piccolo just a few rows over. Our Saturday morning pre-concert rehearsals at Jordan Hall finally reveal the true dimension of our sound, for better or worse. Half of the conductor's work at these final rehearsals is to adjust the balance, warning the brass to play more gently, the woodwinds to be crisper, the strings to play as one. Jordan Hall gives a musician tough love. It rewards only quality. It is a fine instrument, and we as an orchestra have to tune to it.

New Baton

For the next few years, from the middle 1980s to the early 1990s, the orchestra honed its skills and learned to be an ensemble. Over time, it seemed that Maestro Kula's vision for his career and our vision for the orchestra were no longer in sync. Some of the works he programmed seemed more designed to beef up his resume than to best showcase the orchestra. He scheduled difficult works like Stravinsky's *Petrouchka* and Prokofieff's Fifth Symphony that required the hiring of several extra instruments and which, technique-wise, were not what a young nonprofessional orchestra was easily capable of playing. Musicians began to develop musical bad habits—not paying attention to finer dynamic details, "faking" difficult passages, and approximating intonation. The problem went even deeper. Musicians working that hard on their own basics stop listening to one another. They are no longer an ensemble, an organic whole. And the conductor becomes nothing more than a traffic cop.

A debate arose about how "professionalized" the group should become. Kula wanted to pack the ensemble with ringers—trained musicians he knew from his conservatory roots. It's all very well to want to build a group's professionalism. But the Longwood Symphony was created as an amateur ensemble of health care professionals, and that's what it wanted to remain. Many of our amateur musicians had had excellent musical training in their pasts, but medical school, research projects, and surgical procedures had gotten in the way. Under the right leadership, the orchestra had the drive and the ability to continue improving its musical level without outside players. Bringing in ringers may even have stunted that drive, since even highly talented amateurs might lose motivation to improve when professionals were getting to play all the plum passages.

We began to sense that something wasn't right. We were committed as an orchestra to playing in Jordan Hall, one of the city's gems. We knew we needed to bring our level of music up to the level of the hall where artists like Yo-Yo Ma, the Juilliard String Quartet, Maurizio Pollini, and others frequently performed. We could hear the difference, and it was a discordance that we wanted to fix ourselves. It was a crossroads moment.

This all came to a head on what was planned as our greatest concert to date. In October 1991, the Longwood Symphony was invited to play a concert titled "Reverence for Life" for the Albert Schweitzer Fellowship as it launched a new game-changing national program of community service. Master cellist Yo-Yo Ma had agreed to be a part of the concert and the symposium that preceded it, organized by Dr. Lachlan Forrow and Judge Mark Wolf, the president and the chair of the board of the Albert Schweitzer Fellowship. While the orchestra members could barely contain their excitement around playing for such a prestigious guest soloist for such an inspirational organization, our conductor seemed not to be as enthused. In fact, he chided Ma for arriving late to a rehearsal when Ma had generously rushed across town to fit in a rehearsal with us between two other performances. This lack of respect was frighteningly embarrassing. It was the last straw. Soon thereafter, the Board informed Maestro Kula that they would not be renewing his contract.

A Higher Calling

Conductor struggles notwithstanding, the concert in October 1991 with Yo-Yo Ma, a joint concert with the Albert Schweitzer Fellowship, proved to be a watershed moment for us. The concert was the finale of a two-day symposium sponsored by the Harvard Pilgrim Health Care Foundation, and organized by ASF president, Dr. Lachlan Farrow amd ASF chair Judge Mark Wolf.

The idea for the symposium, titled "Reverence for Life" after Dr. Schweitzer's visionary philosophy, was to raise awareness in our community about issues that might have been addressed by Schweitzer himself in the 21st century. Starvation and tropical diseases were not the issues in Boston, but the city had serious issues of its own. For two days, community leaders took over public spaces all over the city to consider four public health challenges: HIV/AIDS, Homelessness, Children's Health, and Domestic Violence. We also discussed Dr. Schweitzer's ethic of Reverence for Life and Schweitzer's views on the music of Bach. The symposium culminated in the LSO's concert at Jordan Hall with soloists Yo-Yo Ma; my husband, violinist Lynn Chang (my husband and a founding member of the Boston Chamber Music Society); and his own violin student Steven Frucht, who was then a Harvard medical student and is now a distinguished neurologist in New York City. It was to be an opportunity to bring together the doctors and staff of the many health agencies who had gathered for the symposium. In addition, these clinics invited patients and clients to attend the remarkable concert. But we discovered something heartbreaking: although every ticket had been distributed, many of the seats remained unfilled. We had overlooked some crucial considerations: homeless clients could not attend our late-night concert because the shelters closed at 10 P.M. Victims of domestic violence could not attend a public performance, for fear of their safety.

Looking out at the empty seats in the house, the medical musicians onstage were moved. What was poignant were the "pertinent negatives"—that some people were *not* in attendance at the otherwise sold-out concert hall. We noticed that there was something different about the music—granted, we *were* inspired by playing with Yo-Yo Ma—but there was something more. Suddenly we were playing our music with a greater degree of passion—a sense of purpose, a sense of healing. That night we played for those who would have filled those empty seats. Those empty seats impressed on all of us the magnitude of the problems facing our community. And we resolved to do something about it, together, as an ensemble.

That was the moment the LSO Healing Art of Music program was born. Dedicated to those missing in the audience that night, we have since committed ourselves to play every concert to make a difference. We offer one third of each concert hall's tickets at a discounted price to a carefully chosen medical nonprofit organization in our community. During the months preceding each concert, we work closely with representatives from the organization to help make their event a success. We teach them to fundraise around the concert and help get their message publicized. Often, our relationships with many of the organizations continue from then on, for years. Each organization is encouraged to use the concert opportunity to fit its unique mission and articulate its unique needs: some organizations honor their researchers, clinicians, and staff; some establish new health initiatives; and two, Boston's Health Care for the Homeless and Mattapan Community Health Center, used their benefit concerts to launch capital campaigns to build new clinics.

Over the past twenty years, the Longwood Symphony has worked with 38 Boston organizations and helped raise more than a million dollars for the medically underserved of our community. As we did at the very first Albert Schweitzer Fellowship concert, we encourage our partner organizations to bring—along with their Board members and benefactors—the patients who benefit from the programs. Our audiences have included teen mothers who had never heard classical music (Dimock Health Center), bouncy hemophiliac boys (New England Hemophilia Association), Cambodian orphans with their new families (The Sharing Foundation), wheelchair-bound radiation victims (Children of Chernobyl), and devoted college students who gathered to raise funds for cancer, in memory of their classmate (Reid Sacco Memorial Foundation).

Dr. Albert Schweitzer encouraged all to "find your own Lambaréné," to find one's own way to serve. Like Dr. Schweitzer, LSO has found its own unique way to combine music, medicine, and community service right here in Boston. For us, Boston—with all its wealth and poverty; its great institutions of culture, education, and medicine next to sinks of ignorance and violence—but above all the creative soul and the affluence of spirit that unites us as artists and scientists—is the Longwood Symphony's very own Lambaréné.

A New Chapter

In 1992, after a conductor-search season in which we invited a different conductor to lead the orchestra at each of our three concerts, we engaged the talented Venezuelan-born conductor Francisco Noya to take the LSO to the next level. Maestro Noya knew how to build an orchestra from within. Equally importantly, Noya understood deeply the power of music for social change. Born in Valencia, Venezuela, Maestro Noya was a friend and colleague of the founders of Venezuela's legendary *El Sistema* program, which will be discussed in greater detail in later in the book. He embraced the orchestra's dual mission of community service and musical excellence.

Noya's experience proved invaluable. After he left Venezuela, he received his degrees in conducting and composition from Boston University. He then went on to conduct two of the best youth orchestras in the country, the Empire State (New York) Youth Orchestra and the Greater Boston Youth Symphony Orchestra. Noya knew that many of our musicians had put their musical training on the back burner after youth orchestra to pursue their medical careers. He picked us up where we had left off and worked from there. By choosing repertoire that helped LSO musicians get their chops back, he helped us develop as musicians. String ensemble improved by selecting works with increasingly complex counterpoint passages, and string sonority was burnished by choosing works, mainly from the Romantic era, whose harmonies required tight musical collaboration between the sections. To soften the hard edges in the brass, he encouraged them to create new aural colors, which stretched their technique. We learned to listen to each other, and during his tenure with us, Noya helped us develop our own signature Longwood Symphony sound.

A Dual Mission To Match its Dual Citizens

Today, there is an ever-growing number of excellent musicians in healthcare who seek a way to keep their lives in balance. Some promising medical students and residents are even choosing Boston just so they can be in a city that has a medical orchestra of LSO's caliber. The more we attract, the better able we are to choose musicians of ever-higher caliber. And the improving caliber in turn attracts even more applicants. Those who audition to us care as much about their own charity work as they do about playing or medicine. They know that we value their dual passion.

When Maestro Francisco Noya announced in 2003 that he would be stepping down after twelve years, he left the LSO in very good health. Under his leadership, the Longwood Symphony Orchestra had found its identity and was in great musical shape. He remains a mentor and friend to the orchestra. Noya passed the baton seamlessly to another long-time friend of the LSO, Jonathan McPhee, who was also Music Director of the Boston Ballet Orchestra. Over the years, McPhee had watched the growth of the Longwood Symphony's model of community engagement with interest. In an interview with the *Boston Phoenix* in 2004, McPhee explained his decision to take on a nonprofessional orchestra: "Part of the attraction over the years has been the fact that it is such a unique organization of some very serious musicians in there; in fact, there are several people in there who actually at one point or another had to make a decision between a music career and a medical career, and they chose a medical career. But here's a collection of extremely intelligent people—everything from surgeons to anesthesiologists. And they've created an orchestra with a very unique mission, which is, every single concert is a benefit. There's no other orchestra in the United States that does that. And I think that's something that's very important, that they can really offer quality music—which is good for them; it's one of the opportunities for the healers to have a healing experience themselves." I clearly recall McPhee's excitement at his first Board meeting when he exclaimed, "Do you know what you are sitting on? The work you are doing is wonderful. But not only are you doing something remarkable as physicians and musicians, but this model may well be an important part of what will be the future of *all* American orchestras. You have found a unique way for your orchestra to become *relevant to the community.*"

He was right. In June 2007, the League of American Orchestras honored our work with the MetLife Award for Excellence in Community Engagement. We shared the stage with two professional orchestras, the Oakland East Bay Symphony and the Philadelphia Orchestra. The award reaffirmed to us that our commitment to bring music, medicine, and community service together in a single purpose was the right path. But the lessons we learned—about playing beyond the music and for the community—are not limited to an orchestra of medical musicians, but apply to orchestras everywhere.

A LOVING COMMUNITY

In preparing this book, I found myself hosting a reunion of the two founders, the Rev. Dr. Guy Steele Sr. and the Rev. Charles W. Kessler. There were hugs and smiles and the two men told their stories as interweaving lines—just as if they were playing a duet. Two people who so overflowed with the urge to help others that they also found time to start a symphony orchestra—one that has not only survived nearly thirty years but thrived. Having seen how far their brainchild had come in that time, the LSO's two founders seemed very much at peace.

"I think the orchestra today is wonderful," Rev. Kessler said. "It's such a marvelous thing to hear the balance, the fullness of the strings, the quality of the brass, the elegance of the woodwinds. When we were organizing the orchestra, Guy and I were talking about how this whole thing fit into our ministry. I remembered something a pastoral educator once told me. He said it is the task of a minister, when entering a church or community, to support the loving community that exists. And if it doesn't exist, you work to create it—"

Rev. Steele jumped in: "—and you create a community to the point that it no longer is necessary to have you in order to survive."

Kessler continued: "I think of the Longwood Symphony Orchestra as the creation of a loving community in the medical area. What it does today in terms of the charity connections, I think that is a continuation of the thrust of this man's ministry," putting an arm around his musical colleague and friend.

What can I say but amen? But now, let's take a closer look at how that community works in the real world.

PART II

Music, Medicine, and Healing

5

Musician-Physician Modulation

NOW THAT YOU KNOW OUR collective history, it's time to meet more of the individuals of today's Longwood Symphony Orchestra and see how music affects us as doctors, and how medicine affects our music. I've chosen just a handful of stories from the dozens that make up the LSO.

We have a research physician whose medical detective work could fill a season of your favorite TV medical drama. We have a young doctor who uses music as therapy for himself. We have brilliant young man from China who holds degrees from Harvard *and* MIT and yet finds that the LSO fills a powerful need. We have a physical therapist who uses her musical skill at listening to improve the care she gives her patients. And we have an occupational therapist who regards her relationship with her violin like a marriage.

DR. STEPHEN WRIGHT: "WHAT IS THAT INSTRUMENT?"

Let's start with Dr. Stephen Wright. Gray-haired and bespectacled, with a welcoming smile and gentle manner, Dr. Wright could easily fit the role of country doctor. Instead, he's the recently retired beloved Chief of Medicine at Faulkner Hospital, and a Professor of Medicine at Tufts Medical School. Speaking in the same baritone voice as his bassoon, Wright said he owes his medical career in part to a humble wart.

"I always had science curiosity and aptitude and always had a really good sense of how things work. I could look at a broken clock and fix it. My parents were always amazed at that."

When he was in second or third grade he developed a wart on his hand. His parents took him to the doctor and he loved all the shiny instruments and the bracing smell of alcohol (used for sterilizing instruments in those days). "When the doctor asked me what the wart felt like I said, 'An inverted cone.' The doctor said that was right, and he knew exactly what kind of wart I had (a 'common' wart). Afterward he told my parents that I might have an aptitude for medicine. They enrolled me in the Junior Science Explorers Program at the Boston Museum of Science, which was a curriculum they offered on Saturday mornings, and I'm proud to say that I am one of their success stories. It just seemed like I was always headed for a career in medicine."

Wright's parents had a passion for the theatre, and got involved in local productions of Gilbert & Sullivan, exposing the boy to the rich variety of colorful music in the operettas outside of school. "My father, who was the stage manager, knew he had to raise the curtain up at a certain point in the score, so he had to read a little bit of music. He didn't play anything or know anything about music, but he knew that *this* many measures into the overture, the curtain should go up. My mother was a soprano and I still remember when she played one of the fairies in *Iolanthe*. So we were taken to those productions early on."

However, the moment that lit the boy's musical fuse occurred when he was in second grade. His father brought home an LP of the Philadelphia Orchestra playing Rimsky-Korsakov's *Scheherezade*. "It has a legendarily beautiful lyrical bassoon solo in it and I must have listened to that a hundred times. And I thought, 'What *is* that instrument?!?' The sound of the bassoon was just so mesmerizing."

Because of its size, the bassoon is an unlikely instrument for a second grader. Wright's parents started him on violin lessons in grammar school, then switched him to clarinet. "I played clarinet through the ninth grade. They seated me in front of a lovely young woman who was a much better clarinetist than I. She's now my wife. But she was too good on the clarinet. I practiced like mad but couldn't quite catch up with her. I had a very bad, volatile temper and one day when I was practicing a passage of 'Malaguena' that has a very tricky clarinet lick, I got so frustrated I broke my clarinet right over my knee! I went down to the kitchen and told my parents it had rolled off the bed.

"The planets lined up perfectly because now I needed a new instrument. And Hingham High School, bless their heart, owned a bassoon, so I switched to the bassoon that year, and finally I got to make that sound that had mesmerized me as a child. I never went back."

Now an accomplished bassoonist and gastroenterologist, Wright bought his first bassoon (vintage 1910) from his music teacher with money he earned on his paper route. Though it was second-hand, it was a Heckel, a fine German instrument. In 1992, when he could afford a better one, Wright, now Dr. Wright, again went for another Heckel (vintage 1983), which he still plays. It's Saturday morning, time for the dress rehearsal before tonight's concert. Opening the bassoon case, Wright lightly touches each piece and lovingly describes it as "the best made."

Fully assembled, a bassoon looks like a long straight wooden pipe, nearly eight feet in length, folded back on itself once from the bottom, the shape of a tight "J," to make it wieldy. Embracing the length of the pipe is a spiderwork of silver keys and rods that enable players to open and close holes in the pipe beyond what a single set of fingers can reach.

As Wright fits the pieces together, he names them, one by one. "There is the bell, of course, which fits into the aptly named long joint. The bottom, where the fold is, is called the 'boot.' The shorter segment of folded pipe is called the wing joint. It ends at mouth level with a curved metal pipe called a 'bocal.' The double reed slips in here."

Bassoons range from dark brown to mahogany red. Made of sturdy mountain maple, Wright's Heckel leans toward red. It is held upright across the waist, with the weight resting on his thumbs. Wright blows through a small curved mouthpiece that looks like the tail on the letter "Q" which has a double reed similar to the one Dr. Sheldon uses on his oboe, only much larger. The rich basso sound emerges from the bell, which seems to have round wooden lips, like—final letter comparison here—a mouth singing the letter "O."

Most wooden wind instruments eventually "blow out"; the vibrations damage the wood and distort and sour the sound after so many years of playing. "Bassoons," on the other hand, "tend to get more mellow," Wright said, warming to the history of his twenty-five-year-old instrument. "This one was 'voiced' for a German orchestra. They traditionally play sharper, so this one used to play sharp. I had an artisan extend a portion of tubing to slightly lengthen the instrument in an attempt to bring the pitch down slightly."

It's that kind of attention to precision that makes a great musician—and a great physician.

DR. MICHAEL BARNETT:
"SOMETHING YOU CAN'T IGNORE"

An O. Henry–like story comes from another of our oboists, Dr. Michael Barnett, a self-confident intern at the Brigham Women's Hospital, who plays first oboe. He is tall, with short dark cropped hair and intense brown eyes that are often peering above his glasses, as if to get an even sharper focus on whatever it is we are discussing.

Both his parents are doctors—his father a primary care doctor and his mom an anesthesiologist who went into medical administration. Barnett's dad even played the saxophone. "I think he was considered to be pretty good," Barnett said, "—not amazing, but pretty good. His teacher had even wanted him to apply to a music conservatory, but he felt he had to make a choice, and he went into medicine. He owned a Selmer Mark 7 sax, which is a very classic saxophone. There really isn't the equivalent of a Stradivarius in the wind world because wind instruments don't get better when they age. But that saxophone is a classic. Every now and then throughout my childhood he would take it out and honk a little bit on it, just to stay in practice. But he saw that my interest in the oboe was growing as I was approaching my teen years. And one year he said, 'You know what? It's time.' And he *sold* his Selmer Mark 7 to buy my first professional oboe, which cost $5,000."

Natural teenage rebellion caused young Michael to avoid medicine at the outset. "Medicine had always been in my life and I had always thought about it and been fascinated by it, but once this music thing bit me, it sort of went by the wayside. After all, why would I dream of doing the same thing my parents did? I forgot about medicine and got sucked into the arts in high school. I loved to read literature. I thought maybe I'd be an English major, or perhaps a history major."

Things changed during Barnett's freshman year at Yale. "I took introductory biology. The course was taught by one of the worst professors I have ever worked with. He was actually the only Nobel Prize winner at Yale at the time, but he just did not care about the undergraduates. Luckily we had a good textbook and I was completely captivated. I had no idea that biology was so intricate and beautiful and that there was so much happening in every single cell, every single subdivision of a cell, in our bodies. It was just like finding a new amazing author or genre of literature that you've never seen before, volumes that you've never explored. It was very exciting for me . . . and I said, maybe I'll give this pre-med thing a try."

DR. READ PUKKILA-WORLEY:
MEDICAL MYSTERIES, MUSICAL SOLUTIONS

In a 2004 segment of NPR's "Morning Edition,"[1] on the Albert Einstein Symphony Orchestra in the Bronx—another medical orchestra—internist and French horn player Dr. Eliot Moshman was quoted as saying that playing music has helped him appreciate what he calls the art of medicine. "It's a question of communication skills with patients, with other doctors," Eliot Moshman said. "There are a lot of ways to make people feel better, other than giving a cut-and-dried answer and writing a prescription. That's what I would call the *art* of medicine, and it's not fluff."

Dr. Read Pukkila-Worley agrees. He is a specialist in infectious diseases and a cellist in the LSO. With big blue eyes, well-trimmed hair, an easy laugh, and a ready smile, Pukkila-Worley sees the good in anyone and gets along with everyone. I met Pukkila-Worley when he was still a fourth-year medical student touring his future home hospital, MGH, and terribly excited that Boston had its own orchestra for doctors. He was one of the few who managed to still play in the orchestra even during his internship (most musicians take a year or two off during those arduous years). Exhausted when he walked into rehearsals, he always seemed rejuvenated by the end. It seems that music truly is his oxygen.

"People ask me if I think about my patients when I'm playing in the orchestra, but actually it usually goes the other way. When I am playing I become immersed in the music. Yet the next day at the hospital I am usually humming something. It brings calm and peace to my life. Many times on the day after a concert or a rehearsal, I will be hearing wonderful music in my head in a way that certainly benefits me. I can only imagine that if *I* am calmer, then I can take better care of my patients—or at least I like to think so. When I am in need of healing I very often turn to music, and it heals me."

Dr. Pukkila-Worley followed in his parents' musical/medical footsteps. "I got into music because it is a very important part of my family," he said. "My grandfather emigrated with his family at the turn of the last century from a small town in Finland called Pukkila. He emigrated to northern Minnesota. He was a clarinetist and my grandmother was a cellist and a vocalist, and so that love of music was then passed to my mother who is a flutist, and to her sister who is a violinist, and then again to me through the generations.

"My grandfather just loved the composer Sibelius. It was in his blood. When I played the Sibelius Second Symphony and his Karelia Suite with the Longwood Symphony, I heard my grandfather in these pieces. I feel my family and I feel my connection to my family and a personal joy when I get to play that."

FOLLOWING THE FAMILY TRADITION, PUKKILA-WORLEY embraced music as well. But his mom, a flutist-scientist, made one thing perfectly clear to her cello-loving son: "She wasn't going to be that Suzuki Method mother who carries her kid's cello," Pukkila-Worley said, laughing. He recalled that he wasn't so happy about having to lug his own instrument to and from lessons and rehearsals.

"Many children of my generation learned to play string instruments with the Suzuki Method, which includes having children play their instruments together in groups. That social aspect was essential for me in developing a love for the instrument. I was a very unwilling teenager, and the peer pressure of the group was a really important incentive for me in continuing to play. It wasn't until college and, in fact, in medical school, that I developed an independent love for playing. Now, long after I'm grown and in practice, the LSO has allowed me to continue with that."

Dr. Pukkila-Worley is part of an Infectious Disease consult service, which means he is a kind of medical detective, helping the primary team of doctors identify the offending bacterium or virus that is wreaking havoc on a patient's health and diagnosing some of the most perplexing medical mysteries. It's no wonder that we call their department "I.D." for short.

"Infectious Disease is about solving problems, and I like thinking about the patients and putting bits of evidence together to come up with a diagnosis and a treatment plan. That problem-solving aspect of infectious diseases has always attracted me. It is a field that allows one to take observations made by seeing patients and then ask questions about the pathophysiology that underlies what you are seeing in patients. The problem-solving aspect of Infectious Disease has always attracted me. I'm both a physician and a researcher, and I use both skills. I actually am a physician-scientist. I have a laboratory at Massachusetts General Hospital and I do basic science research pathogenesis of infectious disease."

As for music and medicine? "There's definitely a link. I'm from Chapel Hill, N.C., and I have played in their community orchestra before I moved to Boston. It was not an orchestra designed as being part of a medical community, yet fifty percent of the people in the orchestra were part of the medical community! I wonder if some of the analytical qualities of music, the structure of music, the beauty of harmony together appeals to medical professionals and scientists that have to do that on a daily basis. Whether or not we all think from the same parts of our brains in some way, I don't know, but they *are* linked.

"In terms of direct parallels with my career and music, I think that other than being meticulous and being careful as you have to do in medicine and in music. Music is more for me just a source of pure joy than something I have to think about. And I thankfully don't think about medicine when I am playing music because I am so immersed in the music. Even the next day I am humming something. It brings a calm and peace to my life. Many times the day after a concert or a rehearsal, I will be hearing wonderful music in my head in a way that benefits or helps me—I can only imagine if I am calmer, then I can take better care of my patients—or at least I like to think so.

"There is a harpist who visits patient rooms at the Brigham and Women's Hospital and plays in the cancer wards and the intensive care units where people are very sick and the families are there. She just quietly sits with her harp and starts playing. And it fills the air with music . . . and I love music, so I am in tune to this. For me it is so calming and I just feel this kind of peace and I feel my shoulders drop. I imagine that it has the same effect for the patients. I'm sure it does. And in that sense I can imagine the music is helping ease this pain—at least that is how I see it.

DR. ANDREA SPENCER: "THEY LOVED WHAT THEY DID"

Dr. Andrea Spencer and her twin sister Dr. Joanna Spencer both attended Yale as music majors and then became doctors, not only inheriting their parents' dark hair and deep brown eyes but their mutual love of music and medicine. Now a fellow resident in child psychiatry at Massachusetts General and McLean Hospitals, Andrea plays viola with the LSO while her sister, a flutist, is an internal medicine resident at the University of Michigan. Their father has been Chairman of Neurosurgery at Yale Medical School for thirty years, and ran the Yale Epilepsy Program with their mother, a flutist and Professor of Neurology.

"They worked together and loved, loved, *loved* what they did," Spencer recalled.

While in New Haven, Andrea played viola in the Yale Symphony and helped found Musical Cure, a chamber group of medical students that played nursing homes, soup kitchens, and hospitals, much like our "LSO on Call" outreach program does now.

"I came to Boston to be in the LSO," she said. "That, plus the international health focus and the flexible curriculum at Harvard that lets you study what you want. But . . . if you talk to anybody who is interested in music at the Harvard Medical School, they are going to tell you about the Longwood Symphony Orchestra."

SHERMAN JIA: MAKING PEOPLE HAPPY

Born in Chengdu, China, concertmaster Sherman Jia is a handsome, soft-spoken man with closely cropped black hair and dark eyes. An intense, self-directed young man, he came to Harvard with two MIT degrees in engineering and was accepted into the elite Health Sciences and Technology program, a joint program between Harvard and MIT. Jia is a serious violinist and a serious scientist who clearly loves both vocations. He is inquisitive and thoughtful: he will query and allow others to share opinions before forming an opinion of his own. Always respectful, he demonstrates a quiet steely resolve that is never confrontational but leaves no doubt about how he feels. In turn, he engenders the respect of others. In short, he is an ideal collaborative scientist, and an ideal chamber musician—from the principal first violinist's chair.

"Most people talk about how being a musician helps us as physicians. But I like to say that being a physician also makes me think about music differently. In medical school you're trained to think about how you can use science to improve people's lives, either through medicine or through whatever therapies there are. It makes me think about how music can be used to make someone happier. I've been playing solo violin recitals every year at MIT as part of my scholarship program. I love to invite my family, my friends, my teachers and everyone I know within the community to come to the concert. It's a way I can share my passion with my friends and my family." I've attended many of his annual recitals—they rival performances by any conservatory student. A few years ago, Sherman's Harvard cardiology professor gave the students a simple assignment: attendance at Sherman's recital—for credit!

"Music affects my brain in a way I really enjoy. I understand that a lot of it is neurological. But to do something I really enjoy and to share that experience with the audience is really, really cool." Over the last few years, Jia spent much of his time doing remarkable research that combined his engineering and medical skills. Working with doctors at Massachusetts General Hospital, he is trying to figure out the genetic basis for how certain people are naturally able to suppress HIV infection. These people are called HIV Controllers or Long-Term Non-Progressors.[2] They are infected with the AIDS virus, but something about them prevents it from progressing to full-blown AIDS. They have been studied intensively for more than a decade[3] in the hope that a treatment or even a cure could be developed.

"Research consisted of a lot of computation and statistics, so it was perfect for me," he said, "and it certainly seemed like such an interesting and worthwhile project. It was a lot of fun trying to figure out all the nuts and bolts of which genetic variances were associated with resistance to HIV, and tease out the genetic underpinnings of how that works. And as I did it, I started thinking about how much it was like trying to perfect my performance of a piece of music. There is a certain elegance in the correct solution to any problem. In music you want to play a certain piece a certain way. At a certain point it becomes very elegant and all of a sudden it makes sense. And that's how you know you have finally reached the point where you know this is both the technical best you can perform the piece and your clearest personal interpretation. The same is true with a scientific problem. It starts out really hard. You apply all your problem-solving ability, and when you find the solution it should also be quite elegant."

It may not be such a coincidence that the word "practice" applies to both our musical life and our medical life.

Tamara Goldstein: "There Are Strings Attached"

In medicine, sometimes there are miracles, and few members of the LSO have seen as many of these as Tamara Goldstein. A violinist with dark eyes, black hair, and a lithe dancer's physique, Goldstein describes herself as "a feather in the wind" regarding how she came to her careers in music and health care.

When she was eight years old, her life was changed by a knock on the door of her house. A man in white linen suit, whom Goldstein described as looking like Professor Harold Hill in *The Music Man*, was going door to door seeking customers for his musical instrument rental business. Goldstein's mother rented a violin at a dollar a month, and Goldstein has never put it down since.

The wind of fate blew again when Goldstein was a freshman at Boston University and not sure what to declare as her major. She was sitting outside with a look of distress on her face when an older woman walked up to her and asked what the matter was. "I said, 'I have to declare a major, but I don't know which direction to take.' The woman asked 'What do you like?' I said I like violin and painting but I also like the idea of helping others and healing and medicine. She said 'Have you ever heard of occupational therapy? You should write that down as your major.'"

And Goldstein did. She was curious enough to try it. Occupational therapists help patients resume their activities of daily living after injury, illness, or disease. Tamara specializes in the care of the elderly patients, helping her patients adapt to progressive disease processes, regain function after injury, and maximize their quality of life despite the presence of illness.

"I ended up loving it," Goldstein said, and the balance her violin gives her today.

"The orchestra has become one of the most important parts of my life," Tamara Goldstein said. "I once told a physician friend that I was feeling exhausted and that shortly I had to leave for an orchestra rehearsal. He said I should just skip the orchestra rehearsal that night. But I couldn't do it. I'd skip something else, but I'd never skip orchestra. The orchestra becomes part of your nutrition. It feeds you.

"My violin feels like a friend. It's a friend I hope to have until the day I die. Actually, it's more than that. It feels like an extension of me, or even a part of me. It's so deeply rooted in who I am. I really care about the instrument. I have a relationship with it. I once wrote a paper for sociology class in college. The subject was 'How Would You Define Marriage?' I described my relationship with my violin. It's not always fun, it's not always easy. I don't always want to do what it demands of me. But overall it makes me feel happy. It's pleasurable, it's fulfilling, and I feel devoted to it. Even if I don't feel like doing an etude one evening, I'll still dust off the strings before putting it carefully in the case. Yes, like marriage, there are strings attached. Both require respect, patience, effort, commitment, discipline, and, of course, love."

DENISE LOTUFO: A HAPPY MEDIUM

Denise Lotufo, a physical therapist and cellist in the LSO, was lucky enough to grow up during a time of comparatively robust public investment in public arts education. Her public school system in New York introduced kids to stringed instruments when they were in elementary school and at age eleven, young Denise was asked to pick her "ax"—her special instrument.

"I wanted to play the bass and my parents wanted me to play the violin," she recalls, "so we decided to settle for a happy medium, the viola or the cello. I was attracted to the sound of the cello, and the more I began to play the cello, the more I fell in love with it. I really feel all the emotions of the cello. Bach's First Suite is still something I really enjoy. It makes me feel settled. I may come home from work feeling a little bit up in the air, but I take the cello out and play a little bit of that First Suite and everything is okay again."

Dr. Lotufo said that the simple act of listening is key to how she does her job as a physical therapist. "I think that in order to really get down to what ails a patient, you have to get to know them. A lot of the medical disciplines don't allow doctors the time to get to know their patients all that well. I have the luxury to do so because of the nature of physical therapy. Patients often talk during their session, whether they're doing exercise or getting hands-on therapy, so I get to know them a little better. How does that help? Occasionally some little intricate part of their personal history will come out that you can use to help them. In chatting, they may share a piece of information they may not have given their physician."

When it comes to the doctor-patient relationship, connection is key. But, as we all know, it can be hard to articulate how we feel. Words like "hurt" or "sore" or "tired" can mean any number of nuanced things. But how can a patient communicate that? How can a physical therapist "read" that? A physical therapist like Lotufo relies more than anyone on the physical senses. Call it "healing hands" or "the healing touch."

She must listen to a patient's tone of voice, see the patient's facial expression, feel through her fingertips how the patient's muscles tighten or relax. Unless your eyes and ears and hands are aware in the right way to all the patient's signals, there is no way to diagnose or heal the whole patient.

"Example: I have a patient who is a runner who used to have constant knee pain when they were running. So we began to treat it like a running injury. But as I was working with them and talking with them, I learned that they also got the pain while just sitting. It ended up not being a joint injury at all, but what we call a 'referral' from their back, meaning that the nerve is registering pain from one part of the body in another part. We were able to give the appropriate treatment simply because I listened.

"When I'm playing cello in the LSO I have to listen carefully all the time. You learn to listen whether you're sharp or flat and when you're playing a note in tune. That helps me listen for the right information from the patient. In both cases, you learn to weed out what's noise and what's not."

One of the more interesting stories is told by one of Denise's patients, seventy-eight-year-old Anne Gamble. Mrs. Gamble volunteers in the chaplain's department at Boston's Children's Hospital, and has always had a deep love of music. It was her secret dream to play the cello, but she was told early in life that her hands were too small to manage the large instrument, a "technical deficiency" that meant she could never achieve her dream. It was a sad thing to learn, but she dealt with the disappointment stoically. She found an outlet for her musical soul by singing in a local choir, and she put her dream on the shelf for nearly seven decades.

When she was seventy-one she began suffering shoulder and neck pain and was referred to physical therapist Denise Lotufo for physical/manual therapy. "There was a very small picture on her wall of someone with a cello," Mrs. Gamble said. "So I asked her why, and she said she played cello in the Longwood Symphony Orchestra. I told her I had always loved classical music and especially loved the sound of the cello. I said that maybe in my next life, I would have long, strong fingers so I could play the cello too. But Denise said I didn't have to wait that long. She suggested that I try playing a seven-eighths size cello. I didn't know they came in different sizes!"

Lotufo directed her to a store in Boston where she could find just the right instrument. Her hands (which to Lotufo seemed perfectly normal-size) finally hefted the instrument that was not too big, not too small, but just right. She described the experience as "heavenly."

Mrs. Gamble start taking lessons, and her teacher organized eight of her students into a cello choir. "She picks challenging music and divides it into two parts so we play, four and four. We've even done some tangos, which are really fun."

For Mrs. Gamble, the advantage of having a musician as a physical therapist was pretty obvious. "I would not be playing cello now if it were not for Denise. During that time she has not only helped me with my shoulder and neck problems so that I really don't have them much anymore, she's also become a very good friend."

The physical activity associated with cello playing may even have helped with that. Proper exercise is often the right therapy, whether it be swimming, stretching—or cello playing. And how does the experience of playing the cello live up to her expectation? "I just love it," she said, beaming. "I just don't feel alive unless I have music."

Mrs. Gamble may have used the expression "feel alive" in a spiritual sense, but we are beginning to understand more and more how, physiologically, playing and listening to music can have a powerful tonic effect throughout the body.

DR. SUSAN PAUKER: "WE'VE TRIED EVERYTHING"

And now, a story of struggle and transcendence. Dr. Susan Pauker is Chief of Medical Genetics at Harvard Vanguard Medical Associates. As such, she sometimes has to shoulder the unenviable task of delivering bad news to people who least expect it and are sometimes least prepared to absorb it.

A highly regarded physician whose friendly face and bright blue eyes reflect years of compassion and experience, Dr. Pauker speaks of life-and-death issues with a steady voice, touched with a quiet sense of urgency, and always with empathy. "I may diagnose an abnormality of a fetus, and then I help the family decide if they are continuing the pregnancy. Or I diagnose a father with Huntington's disease and I have to talk to his daughter, a young woman who just had a baby, about the fact that she and the baby are at risk and does she want them to be tested. So every day, all day long, it is really, really, *really* intense."

Dr. Pauker crisscrosses Longwood Avenue throughout the week because her services are in demand: she is on the staff at Massachusetts General Hospital, practices Medical Genetics at Harvard Vanguard in Kenmore, and teaches as Associate Professor of Pediatrics at Harvard Medical School. She also heads the august Francis Weld Peabody Society, one of the four "houses" that divide Harvard Medical School a bit like Harry Potter's Gryffindor House, et al., at the mythical Hogwarts School of Witchcraft and Wizardry. The mission of the real-life Peabody Society is nothing less than "to create and nurture a diverse community of the best people committed to leadership in alleviating human suffering caused by disease."

As co-Master, Pauker mentors medical students to find ways to accomplish Peabody Society's mission and to individualize it to whatever medical specialty they choose. She teaches them about academics, clinical work and work-life balance, including music.

Pauker trained at Massachusetts General Hospital as a pediatrician with some studies in genetics. As the field began to explode, thanks to new technology and research in the 1970s and 1980s, she shifted all of her work to genetics and including the study of syndromes and birth defects, including autism, Down syndrome and Marfan syndrome. She said, "The kind of stuff I had to do with patients became incredibly more complex." She counsels patients to make some of the most difficult decisions of their lives.

Dealing with the impact of these sorts of difficult decisions is not unfamiliar to Sue and Stephen Pauker. Pauker's husband has cerebral palsy, the result of a brain injury he suffered when he was born with the umbilical cord wrapped around his neck. When he was a child, his parents were told to institutionalize him because he would be retarded. They didn't. Susan Pauker, his wife of nearly fifty years, relishes telling the capper to the story: "When he graduated *first in his class* at Harvard Medical School, the Cerebral Palsy Society of Kingston, NY wrote 'Oops.'" Stephen is now a prominent cardiologist and a professor at Tufts medical school. He counts among his patients the legendary Arthur Fiedler, conductor of the Boston Pops.

Though not a musician himself, Stephen loves music. "Here he is with zero coordination," Pauker laughs. "It's a real challenge for him to walk. And yet musicals like *West Side Story* and *My Fair Lady* make this man crazy with happiness."

Music may be a genetic legacy in Pauker's family. Her last name means "drummer" in German. "Music is kind of a holy thing for me," Dr. Pauker said. "It's very spiritual. When I talk to patients about medication, I also talk about seeking the help of a higher power, whatever that might be for them. Patients with genetic disorders often experience chronic pain. They dislocate everything they own and everything hurts all the time and it's going to get worse and there's no treatment. I do strongly recommend medication for people in chronic pain. But I also recommend hypnotherapy. I recommend meditation. I recommend Tai Chi—and I recommend music. I don't prescribe any particular piece or even any particular kind of music. If you can soak in a hot tub because that seems to bring healing and play the music that you love and have that be your ten minutes the kids can't come in—then that's how it ought to be.

"It helps me to do my job. It refills my tank in a way that allows me to give to patients. I give *all* day long, *all* day long, *all* day long to advise medical students or care for the patients, and this is a chance for me to receive healing. When we played at my mom's assisted-nursing home, she and all her friends there were crying because they were so moved. They said, 'Come back tomorrow.' That was a big deal. That's healing. That's giving. So is making a difference to a charitable organization that is serving the underserved. I feel like practicing *becomes* my community service. It is giving. That is how it feels to prepare music that's going to raise money for an organization, especially when it is one that is precious to me—like when we did the concert for the March of Dimes, because they help people prevent birth defects. When our work of playing benefits another group, it's got this gigantic secondary gain."

Her love for music and for being part of the LSO is deep. But Dr. Pauker has a difficult secret. She reaches behind her blond tresses that fall on either side of her head and pulls two objects from her ears. She tosses them down in sad anger.

Hearing aids. Pauker is gradually losing her hearing and is already functionally deaf without them.

"I've been identifying with Beethoven," she said. "I had some sort of accident in a dental office about two years ago—something to do with the high-pitched sound of the drill. We know that my 'organ of Corti,' the tiny structures in the ear that convert vibrations to nerve impulses, was damaged, but we still don't really understand how that happened. I'm surrounded with some of the top doctors in the world, but no one has been able to help. We've tried everything—injected intra-cochlear steroids, everything. But it's gone. I don't really have much hearing now.

"I've got these two little toys that help me hear," she continued, pointing to her hearing aids, "and I've also taken courses on how to position yourself and watch faces. I even have a little receiver in my office for when patients are crying or sad and are speaking quietly so I have a chance of hearing what they are saying without asking them to repeat it." She pauses and sighs. "It's pretty tragic."

Dr. Pauker said she uses a variety of strategies to deal with her problem. In addition to the hearing aids, she said she watches the conductor more attentively than most. Seated on the left side of the stage in the second row of violins, she is able to take her cue by watching the way the bows of the first-row violins move.

She also relies on her stand partner. "The conductor will say 'Let's start at C.' For me, 'C' could be Z or D or B. I have no clue what he's saying. Every once in a while he'll remember to say 'C for Cat' or 'D for David' for the benefit of the musicians in the back, and that helps me. My stand partner hears well and as soon as Jonathan says anything he points with his bow. He's just divinely accommodating. I never have to ask him, he just automatically does it."

So why doesn't Dr. Pauker just quit? Because she loves it. It is simply her love of the music and the strong role it plays in her life.

"One thing about physicians," she said, "we have to be really, really competent. We have to be right at the top of our game. You can't just look in a patient's ear and say everything's okay. You have to be thinking: Could it be this? Could it be that? In pediatrics I felt that I could glide on my knowledge some weeks and not be reading the latest article. In genetics you have to be right at the top of your game. You have to be doing research as you practice because things are changing so fast. And competent is what we are."

Pauker says the music is necessary to her own health. "When you say 'What does music *mean* to you?' I can't even begin to tell you what it means to me." Later, she says "Certain moments in music give me life. We played Gershwin's *Rhapsody in Blue* in summer 2010 and I love the parts where it gets rich and huge. When I'm inside something so spectacular like that and I know it so well, I still really feel that I am contributing. It was wonderful. But when the music is delicate and little and fast and you really need to rely on hearing, I . . . I . . . I . . . don't know if I should continue. I think maybe I should stop. The orchestra has gotten better and better and better . . . and I'm not getting better. I'm scared to death. I can't tell whether I am being selfish. That's what scares me.

"I don't usually pray. I've prayed for patients and I've prayed out of gratitude. But when we played at Tanglewood last summer, I prayed because I *didn't want to screw up*. I had promised myself that if I screwed up, it would be my last concert. At the dress rehearsal I played an extra note I wasn't supposed to play, and all afternoon before the performance I was devastated because we were going to record the performance that night and I afraid I was going to damage it. The oath we take as doctors is *'Primum no nocere'*—'First, do no harm,' and I was just demolished emotionally that day because I was worried I was going to harm the performance and the recording. I thought, 'This is it. This is the *last time I am playing.*' That's when I prayed to not do harm. And then it turned out fine. The conductor was happy with the recording. And I thought, 'Okay, I'm still good enough to continue. Occasionally I can still make a nice rich contribution.'"

These days, there is a lot of public discussion about the need for clinicians to return the humanity and humanism to the field of medicine. Dr. Pauker's compassion for her patients, medical students, and colleagues is legendary. There is no doubt about how much she will contribute to the heart—and the soul—of the LSO.

6

Music As Healing

MUSIC MAY HAVE POWER TO soothe the savage beast, but does it have any actual power to heal the body? Everyone knows sickness in the body can cloud the mind, and sickness in the mind can affect our physical health. Less well known is how beneficial input like music can make us well—or, at any rate, better.

You leave work at the end of a long day. Whether you like your work or not, you're tired. Physically tired and mentally tired. You get out the door of your office building or you get behind the wheel of your car or you climb on a bus or you shut down whatever loud machinery you've been operating all day, and the first thing you do is click on the radio . . . or pop in the earbuds and thumb through to your favorite song . . . or perhaps you just sing softly to yourself.

Even before you eat dinner, you crave music. The tunes, the beat, the harmony—each song has a special highlight. Even reading this now, you can't help running your mind over a favorite song.

There are chords and passages in music we lean into, like a cat leaning into your hand when you pet it. For some it's the "Ode to Joy" passage in Beethoven's majestic Ninth Symphony. For others its Eric Clapton's guitar solo on the original recording of "While My Guitar Gently Weeps," the harmonies in "Edelweiss" from *The Sound of Music,* or the beautiful largo movement of Gershwin's *Rhapsody in Blue* (written, incidentally, on a train trip to Boston).

Why? Because music makes you feel better. It works fast and it works nearly every time. The mind lifts. If you didn't know better, you'd say music actually calms your heartbeat and relaxes your muscles. In fact, that's exactly what happens. And that's only the palpable effect. New research is showing that music also acts as a tonic in subtle ways all over the body. It's not just one of today's newest trends: it has been practiced for such a long time and has found proponents among so many serious scientists in the field. Music *is* medicine.

Then why has medical science made so little use of a force that has such immediate and obvious benefits? The study of music's effect on health is garnering more and more interest as a science, but the impact of music is hard to quantify. Even if we document a patient's response to music, noting a decrease in blood pressure, a relaxation of tight muscles, or reflief of headache, we are only scratching the surface. Music simply does not fit easily into the scientific model.

EARLY MUSIC THERAPY

As I described in Chapter Three, music has been utilized as a therapy in many cultures since mankind's earliest days. Chinese medicine recorded its use five millennia ago.[1] Indian Ayurveda ("Science of Life"), developed two thousand years ago, found benefits in chanting still used today in the practice of yoga.[2] The soothing, rhythmic qualities of music have long been judged to have therapeutic qualities for body and mind, but based primarily on intuition and anecdotal experience. The history of music therapy since the Industrial Revolution of the mid nineteenth century has been the story of a quest for ways to turn those instinctive feelings into a real science. Researchers were convinced that benefits seemed so palpable there had to be a way to measure and classify them and thereby calibrate the application of music as a therapy.

Systematic scientific research began with researchers simply seeking to learn what kinds of music could help which kinds of patients and which kinds of illnesses under what conditions. According to the American Music Therapy Association's official history, the first published article about Music Therapy was "Music Physically Considered," an unsigned article published in *Columbian Magazine* in 1789. Research by Dr. Benjamin Rush at the turn of the nineteenth century produced two medical dissertations that dealt with treating disease with music, then using the only delivery system available to them: live musicians.

But controlled research took off with Thomas Edison's late 1800s invention of the phonograph, which enabled large numbers of subjects to be tested with the same pieces of music played the same way. In 1899, Dr. James Coming of New

York connected patients to the phonograph with rudimentary headphones and used a hood to block out extraneous sights and sounds while the music played. He found not only that "large areas of the cerebrum were beneficially affected" by music, but that the benefits accrued whether or not the patient was conscious.[3]

Early twentieth century experiments with both animals and humans showed that music could effect "changes in cardiac output, respiratory rate and volume, pulse rate, blood pressure, and body secretions related to various types of music."[4]

In 1914 the Journal of the American Medical Association published its first letter on the subject. Dr. Evan O'Neill Kane reported using a phonograph during surgery for "calming and distracting patients from the horror of the situation."[5]

These early scientific studies excited a great deal of exuberance about the budding field. In 1917, Eva Vescelius, founder of the National Therapeutic Society of New York City, predicted, "When the therapeutic value of music is understood and appreciated, it will be considered as necessary in the treatment of disease as air, water and food."[6]

The following year, Margaret Anderton, a British musician who had worked with wounded soldiers in World War I, began teaching "Musicotherapy" at Columbia University in New York.[7] She based her teachings on research into whether specific types of music, specific passages in music, and even specific chords could be used to treat specific maladies. Subsequent research found that such claims overreached.

With music therapy studies and practices springing up throughout the Western world, several attempts were made to create professional organizations that would standardize practices, offer peer review to research, and publish scholarly journals. In 1903, the previously cited Eva Augusta Vescelius founded the National Society of Musical Therapeutics. Isa Maud Ilsen founded the National Association for Music in Hospitals in 1926. Harriet Ayer Seymour founded the National Foundation of Music Therapy in 1941. None of these organizations lasted.[8]

Modern Music Therapy

The modern history of Music Therapy as a science began during World War II, when members of the Musicians Emergency Fund visited hospitals that tended vets suffering from what was then known as "shell-shock," now known as Post-Traumatic Stress Disorder, or PTSD. PTSD is defined by the National Institute of Mental Health as "an anxiety disorder that some people get after seeing or living through a dangerous event. . . . People who have PTSD may feel stressed or frightened even when they're no longer in danger." Symptoms include panic attacks and flashbacks in which patients believe they are reliving the trauma over and over. PTSD can affect anyone who has gone through a trauma, and much has been written about Vietnam War veterans suffering from the disorder. But apparently PTSD has affected veterans as long as there have been wars.

Doctors in the 1940s noticed that even the most withdrawn and deeply traumatized soldiers reacted readily and positively to the sound of familiar tunes.

Dr. Suzanne B. Hanser, the founding Chair of the Music Therapy Department at Berklee College of Music, and a leading researcher in the field, said, "Men who were not responding to other treatments—some who were completely unable to speak—would sing along or suddenly say, 'My mother used to sing that to me.'" Music is that powerful and since then, medicine has utilized music as therapy in other health settings outside the arena of war.

"The Violin Doc"

Dr. Mary Rorro is a psychiatrist trained at Massachusetts General Hospital who now works at a Veterans' Administration Hospital in New Jersey. Her sessions with veterans combine conversation with music—with Dr. Rorro herself performing on the viola. While she admits that this is not Music Therapy in the strict sense, she has observed that listening to the music seems to allow the patients to access deeper feelings and speak more openly about the effects of Post-Traumatic Stress Syndrome. "Over the last five years, the VA has nearly doubled the amount of music therapists it keeps at its clinics," she wrote. "Despite the lack of agreement about the effectiveness of music therapy, a recent study found certain parts of a person's brain are triggered when the person listens to music they find enjoyable."[9, 10]

"I wanted to be a doctor since I was four years old," she said. "It was in my blood, and I was committed to it! My father was a general practitioner and his office was in the house, so I saw patients coming and going all the time. A number of my uncles were also doctors, as was an aunt (one of three female physicians I knew at the time).

"I started the violin when I was six and a half years old with the Suzuki method. My mother played with me, and I have such wonderful memories of playing with my mom.

Sometimes we'd play outside and I have memories of playing my violin in the fresh air, listening to the birds.

"As I grew up, I volunteered as a candy striper. I played for patients even then. There was a man who had cancer who was extremely depressed. After I played for him, he started to speak again. The nurses couldn't stop talking about it. I started the viola at fifteen years old and after a while gave up the violin completely because I loved the rich sound of the viola so much more. I majored in music at Bryn Mawr. I was president of the orchestra and principal of the viola section, although I still knew that I was going to medical school.

"I became a psychiatrist [Harvard Psychiatry program, McLean and Massachusetts General Hospital and started the 'A Few Good Notes' program for vets with other employees from the VA Hospital. It has grown into a national program around the country. I found that there were musicians at other VA hospitals all the way to Guam and out West who are interested in playing music for the vets. They get together and play for the patients, usually around the holidays.

"The veterans have found it very therapeutic. There are some who open up and speak after I've played for them and when I see them in the hall, they ask when I'll be playing for them in session again. I have my viola in my office all of the time, and sometimes I play for them in their individual therapy sessions as well. It creates an empathic environment. Every year I also play at the WWII memorial in Washington, and I used to play in the VA Medical/Musical group in Washington DC that performs annually on Veterans Day."

Despite her instrument, Dr. Rollo has earned a nickname from the patients: "The Violin Doc."[11]

MUSIC THERAPY VS. MUSIC MEDICINE

This debate brings us back to Dr. Hanser at Berklee, who co-authored the book *Manage Your Stress and Pain Through Music* with Dr. Susan Mandel, and is past president of both the World Federation of Music Therapy and National Association for Music Therapy. She lectures around the world, and has published research in journals of multiple disciplines. In 2002, she was named by the Boston Globe as one of eleven "People Changing the World" and has been named winner of the 2012 "Lifetime Achievement Award" from the American Music Therapy Association.

She differentiates between Music Therapy and Music Medicine. According to the American Music Therapy Association (AMTA, 2008), "Music therapy is the clinical and evidence-based use of music interventions to accomplish individualized goals within a therapeutic relationship by a credentialed professional who has completed an approved music therapy program"(A). Music medicine, on the other hand, is "typically used by medical personnel (non-music therapists, such as physicians, nurses, dentists, and allied health professionals) as an adjunct to various medical treatments or situations. It often represents an attempt to provide a non-pharmacological intervention for stress, anxiety, and/or pain for the medical patient. [B (Dileo, 1999) p. 4]

As early as 1946, Dr. E. Thayer Gaston began teaching music therapy at the University of Kansas and authored the seminal book *Music in Therapy* and helped found the National Association for Music Therapy in 1950. He advocated finding musicians and giving them training in psychotherapy.

At Pacifica college, Wilhelmina Harbert established a clinic for significantly developmentally delayed people and began to apply the same music therapy principles. She got many of the same results. Children who had trouble learning in traditional ways were able to learn through memorizing little songs and chants, learning simple concepts like right and left the way we use the alphabet song to learn our ABCs. Children who couldn't verbalize at all were shown that they could make music with simple instruments.

But after the 1960s, further advances in the field were stymied by an increasing demand in society and in scientific circles for quantifiable proof. And it was true that music's impact on health could not be observed under a microscope or measured with a blood test.

In 1986, Dr. Jayne M. Standley of the Center for Music Research at Florida State University published a sweeping examination of research up to that time, "Music Research in Medical/Dental Treatment: Meta-Analysis and Clinical Applications," which sorted out which early systematic studies had yielded statistically significant results, and which had not. She found that the effects of music are often small—sometimes less than three percent difference—but measurable. Virtually all the studies showed some improvement in various types of patients thanks to music. She found that pulse rate was affected the most, while length of labor was affected the least.

Another meta-analysis, "Music for Pain Relief," published in Cochrane Review by The Cochrane Collaboration in 2006, cautioned that the effects of music are small and music alone should not be relied upon for pain relief.[12]

Nevertheless, it was clear that music was stimulating certain regions of the brain. The field acquired its equivalent of a microscope in the early 1990s with the development of

Functional Magnetic Resonance Imaging, known as fMRI. This technology has given new impetus to the field, and works in a clever way. As we breathe, oxygen enters our blood stream and attaches itself to a substance called hemoglobin. We know that when areas of the brain are activated, they require greater bloodflow to deliver more oxygen, thus a greater inflow of hemoglobin, like a fleet of delivery trucks. fMRI works on the premise that oxygen-poor hemoglobin react differently in a magnetic field than oxygen-rich hemoglobin. The fMRI picks up on these changes of oxygen levels to create a three-dimensional picture of what parts of the brain are more active during certain activities—activities like playing music or listening to music.

The fields of music therapy, neuroscience, psychiatry, and medicine began to come together, thanks to this new imaging modality. The field enjoyed advances from several distinguished proponents and researchers. One was Dr. Anne J. Blood, now Assistant Professor of Psychiatry at Harvard Medical School and a psychiatric research scientist in the Department of Neurology at Massachusetts General Hospital. She helped develop the technology that allows us to see brain activity when people are listening to music. That technology has found a wide range of uses in diagnosing brain malfunctions.

Using some of that same technology, Dr. Blood and Dr. Robert Zatorre of McGill University in Montreal did research into how the brain responded specifically to music. Their subjects listened to pieces of music that gave them chills, and we learned that music operated in many of the same centers of the brain that were activated by food, sexual activity, and psychoactive drugs. They found that they all stimulate the brain to release the chemical dopamine, one of the substances that enable brain cells to communicate with each other, and which imparts a sensation of intense pleasure. When the Associated Press covered one of their scholarly papers[13] published in the journal *Nature Neuroscience*, the headline read, "To your brain, music is as enjoyable as sex."

In another paper, "Songs of Experience: Music and the Brain," Dr. Zatorre wrote, "Music sometimes has apparently miraculous effects on patients with nervous system damage. For decades, the clinical literature has documented examples of aphasia patients who, suffering from a lesion in the left frontal or superior temporal lobe, can sing fluently but have almost entirely lost the ability to speak. Other isolated reports have described people with advanced senility who have forgotten even their own family, but may be able to remember tunes and lyrics. The fact that these abilities can be readily engaged by music suggests that these functions are not entirely lost, and could potentially be restored. Understanding how music naturally brings these capacities back online in the brain could lead to new therapeutic strategies for neurodegeneration and brain damage."[14]

At last, we had hard physiological evidence of the power of music.

Fortunately, Dr. Hanser was at hand just at the moment when these new tools became available. She elegantly combined her clinical knowledge, developed over many years, with the new technology. She was appointed to the Zakim Center for Integrative Therapies at Dana-Farber Cancer

Institute, where she has done research on the effects of music in the metastatic breast cancer chemotherapy unit, and where she confirmed that it has small but measurable therapeutic effects

"Music therapy has the potential to invoke a new order of healthcare," she said, "one where patients enter the medical center not just to be passively treated and cured, but also to activate their own creative capacity to take control of their health. Music therapy interventions are sometimes so simple and obvious that they may not be taken seriously, even though there is a reasonable amount of scientific evidence to support many of these strategies. Consider the woman who, during a dreaded blood draw, sang the song we wrote together and felt no pain. I recall meeting a frightened young boy entering the medical center and, a week later, witnessed him fighting his discharge because he hadn't finished the music video he was creating in music therapy. And then there's the gentleman who awoke from major surgery to the sounds of the Native American flute, and showed the most stable vital signs the post-op team had ever seen."

MUSIC AND WORK

Work songs are some of the oldest kinds of "pop" songs, which is to say they are known and sung by everyday people rather than professional musicians. They are usually strongly rhythmic to help the workers, whether they are field hands or sailors, to accomplish their tasks in a coordinated way at a greater speed than they might accomplish it if each person worked at their own pace.

Modern office workers don't often have to pull together in quite the same way, though many rely on iPods, radios, and

Muzak to soothe and focus them as they go about their business. But there is one place other than the dance hall where
today's people like to hear something with an insistent beat
to help them with purely physical effort: the gym. Modern
health clubs pipe in music that is not too distracting, yet keeps
the customers on the stair machines, the treadmills, and the
resistance machines pumping away. But does it really help?

In a 2009 British study, twelve male students were asked
to ride stationary bicycles for twenty-five minutes while listening to pop music. They performed this on three separate
occasions, unaware that the researchers increased the tempo of
the music by ten percent on one occasion and decreased it by
ten percent on another. The results showed that they worked
harder, covering a greater virtual distance at a greater virtual
speed, when the music played faster. They worked less hard
and covered less virtual ground when the music was slower.
Moreover, they told the researchers that they liked the music
faster even though it made them work harder and caused more
physical strain/taxation.[15]

Health Magazine wrote about classes in MTACB, Music
Therapy-Assisted Childbirth, in which music was used at all
stages of birth, from the late-prenatal period through labor pains,
contractions, delivery, the postnatal minutes, and even through
early breastfeeding to make the entire experience calmer and less
painful (and for both parents!).[16] Called "Soundbirthing," the
technique was developed and taught by certified doula (labor
assistant) Marie Bigelow in Boise, Idaho, and includes teaching
future parents how to write their own lullabies.

USA Today reported on a series of studies finding that
music actually has a general ability to decrease pain throughout

life. The most recent of the studies, originally published in the *Journal of Advanced Nursing,* tracked sixty patients with chronic pain. Listening to an hour of music on headphones each day resulted in "significantly less pain and depression and an increased sense of control."

The study's authors, Sandra Siedlecki of the Cleveland Clinic and Marion Good of Case Western Reserve, offered several theories for the reduction in pain, including the possibility that music affects hormones or the immune system via the brain. Siedlecki allowed that it "obviously has something to do with mind–body interaction," but speculated that the effect could be as simple as "a pleasant, but powerful, form of distraction." [17]

As far back as 2001, researchers found that surgical patients listening to music such as harp, piano, orchestras, or slow jazz suffered less post-surgical pain. [18]

Bridging the Body and the Mind

Making music was one of the first skills that made us human. Among the earliest relics of mankind's distant ancestors are delicate flutes made from the bones of birds. Instruments of hide and wood may also have existed at this time, but may simply not have survived the predations of time. Chanting and playing drums remain a part of nearly every culture, from the most primitive to the most developed.

Everyone makes fun of waiting room music. But it is designed to be a kind of all-purpose relaxation medicine before you even see the doctor. There's even a word for such all-purpose medicines: *panacea*—and music may have been the first of them.

Music is certainly not the only sensory stimulus that makes us feel better. The smell of fresh flowers, the sight of a handsome man or a beautiful woman, the touch of a loved one's hand—all of them can produce dopamine and other chemicals that signal pleasure and that the brain uses to reward itself. Other positive pursuits like yoga, exercise, and favorite hobbies combine to produce these chemicals.

If music can make you feel better, can music also make you feel bad? Store owners in Minneapolis used our beloved classical music to drive away loitering gang members. Police and transit officials in Portland, Oregon did the same to chase petty criminals away from a transit hub.[19]

But the upsetting power of music, specifically, can go beyond simply annoying people who don't like a certain type of music. During World War II, the Luftwaffe attached piercing sirens to dive bombers during its blitzkriegs to terrify and disorient its victims as it attacked then. When Panamanian dictator Manuel Noriega barricaded himself in the Vatican's Embassy in Panama, the U.S. military smoked him out by blasting loud rock music into the compound until he and his entourage finally fled.

Why Your Brain Likes Music

One of the most fascinating and brilliant members of the LSO is Dr. Psyche Loui, an instructor in neurology at the Beth Israel Deaconess Medical Center at Harvard Medical School. She is a beautiful Chinese-Canadian woman with long black hair, expressive hands, and brown eyes that always seem to be questioning. When she starts to explain a complex neurologic concept such as the neural pathways involved in perceiving sound, she gets a faraway look in her eyes as though she herself is traveling through the brain from synapse to synapse. She plays violin for us, and her special area of research happens to be music and the brain.

There is a question I've always wondered about—a question that is incredibly obvious and yet very rarely considered. Is the response to music purely emotional, or is it physical as well? In other words, is there some actual physical, measurable change that takes place in the body when listening to music? I was certain that if any of my colleagues knew the answer, it would be Dr. Loui.

"I think emotional connection probably has a physical underpinning," she said. "There are several theories: One of my favorites comes from Leonard Meyer, who wrote a book called *Emotion and Meaning in Music* in 1956, positing that music arouses emotion by a slight violation of expectation. If you hear sounds that you completely expect, then it is totally boring and you would not like it. Conversely, if you hear something that is so odd that it seems to come from the middle of nowhere, then you would also not like it. There is something about systematically violating these expectations—something in the middle—that is just right. There are a lot of brain-imaging and brain-physiology studies looking at what kind of things people 'expect' to hear. Our expectations are very strong. If you hear a piece that starts in C major you 'expect' it to end in C major. If it ends in F-sharp major instead, you would say it sounds wrong. And even people with no musical training could tell you that, and would show the brain signatures and physiological signals in response to this type of expectations. Expectations are also found in language: for instance, if someone says 'I take my coffee with cream and . . .' you would not expect to the sentence to end with 'socks.'

"These are violations of expectations at the mind level that you can measure with physiological signals that have very clear brain correspondence."

Our expectation of what comes next is always being teased. Music is full of little moments when expectations are evoked and then frustrated or fulfilled on a very deep level. It's part of the magic of music, and how sound can stir our emotions. A dissonant sound bothers us; when the dissonance resolves, we get that nice 'ahh' moment of sinking into the resolving chord. We may not know a resolving chord from an umbilical cord, but our brains somehow do, and they respond with amazing consistency across ages, genders, and nationalities.

All this takes us back to that even more fundamental question: Why do certain combinations of notes sound good to us at all? "There is a lot of research going on about that," Dr. Loui said, and, interestingly enough, a lot of it involves math. "Music very broadly obeys certain basic mathematical principles. An octave is always two times the frequency of the octave below it. So the orchestra tunes to 440 Hz which is 440 cycles per second of sound vibrations. An octave above that has to be twice that, or 880 Hz. In a Western equal-tempered musical scale, we have a chromatic scale which is twelve logarithmically even divisions of that 2:1 frequency ratio. The reason why we ended up choosing that twelve-note logarithmically even equal tempered musical scale is that the tones that map on to the scale works out quite well as being close to low integer ratios of each other. For instance, a musical interval of a fifth is a 2:3 ratio of frequency. So for example an E is a perfect fifth above A (440), so it is a 3:2 ratio, or 660. Those kinds of ratios have been known since Pythagoras' time to be important for sounds to be consonant together and to sound good."

But where do these expectations, and the math underlying them, come from? From very primal sources: the sounds of nature and the human voice itself.

"The human voice has a certain resonant structure," Dr. Loui said. "When I am talking, there is a certain fundamental frequency to my voice which is about, I'd say, 200 Hz. On top of that, there are all kinds of partials that are whole integer ratios above that. So the ways that sound vibrates in the larynx are actually congruent with the way that musical theory has evolved. There are principles in music theory about what makes music sound good. Music is reflective of physical principles of sounds in the world, especially the human voice."

And, of course, it's not just the various pitches of music that human beings respond to. In his book *This Is Your Brain on Music*, author Daniel Levitin wrote that ". . . most operas, symphonies, sonatas, concertos, and string quartets have a definable meter and pulse, which generally correspond to the conductors movements; the conductor is showing the musicians where the beats are, sometimes stretching them out or compressing them for emotional communication. Real conversations between people, real pleas of forgiveness, expressions of anger, courtship, storytelling, planning and parenting don't occur at the precise clips of a machine. To the extent that music is reflecting the dynamics of our emotional lives, and our interpersonal interactions, it needs to swell and contract, to speed up and slow down, to pause and reflect. . . . The brain needs to create a model of a constant pulse—a schema—so that we know when the musicians are deviating from it."[20]

Just as there are many neural circuits in the brain picking up different sensory information at all times, members of an orchestra function like neurons and each part of the orchestra is responsible for a different part of the music. Similarly, the conductor functions like a corpus callosum that coordinates and integrates the different functions into a single "consciousness." This may be why it is so pleasing to us as musicians to be in an orchestra.

Mystery of Evolution

Of all the skills humans evolved over the eons, the capacity to enjoy music is one of the most mysterious.

"There is a big question about the source and evolutionary progenitors of both music and language," Dr. Loui said. "The probable answer is that they were same thing. Steven Mithen wrote in a book called *The Singing Neanderthals* that music and language both evolved from something that he called 'proto language.' First there was the desire to communicate and the need to form groups. Those are the things that pressured language to develop and also the need to communicate emotions. And the need for language development puts pressure on the brain and on the larynx and the rest of the sound-making physiology. Those kinds of developmental pressures have given us the ability—this extra cognitive, perceptual, and neural ability to make music. Music may have come of that. There is a lot of controversy to that, of course."

Loui quotes evolutionary psychologist Steven Pinker as saying that he thinks music is nothing more than "auditory cheesecake." Needless to say, this statement was very contro-versial—meaning that there is no real evolutionary value to music. After all, as complex as music can actually be, anyone can enjoy it even if they have no idea of exactly what is going on "under the hood," as it were. Dr. Loui continues: "When people hear a modulation, for instance, they may have no idea which key is changing to which or why. They just feel the emotional lift. Or if you're sitting in an audience, you can more or less tell when a song or a symphony is coming to an end. You may not know that the music is headed toward the dominant note or that a chord is about to resolve. But you sense that something is moving the music toward some kind of conclusion.

"There are all these tricks that composers use to play with your expectations," Dr. Loui said, "For instance a coda, or a Picardy third in which a piece in minor suddenly becomes major in the end—it's like suddenly the sun comes out. So there's this one moment when the composer knows he is ful-filling your expectations, and people really enjoy it."

Loui knows more about the mechanics of music than most musicians. Does all that technical knowhow spoil its wonder, like knowing how magicians perform their illusions?

"I don't think so," she said. "I think it's improved it. Knowing how an important structure, let's say the Eiffel Tower, is built, doesn't make it less grand. I think you still appreciate the grandeur of something even if you know how every piece of it was put together. It's a good point, because I find myself going to concerts and analyzing them, using per-ceptual principles and music theoretical principles and saying 'I know why that part was so moving, it was because it just went from minor to major' or it went from very loud to very soft. But I think it makes you just appreciate more the genius of the composer, in knowing that placing that element there at that point will be effective.

"My undergraduate musicology teachers would play a piece by Mozart, and then would add, 'If you were a less important composer, you would have done this other thing.' The 'other thing' would be okay and certainly what you expected to hear, but less soulful and less inspiring. I think knowing the science part doesn't detract from the music part of it."

As an example, Loui described her favorite moment in music. It comes in Beethoven's Ninth Symphony. "There is this very very quiet part in the fourth movement after a loud chorus, where there's a viola solo—go figure! I think that's one of the most hair-raising moments in Western classical music. But I like it a lot."

Most of the things we are, as human beings—the way we look, the way our bodies work, the kinds of things that interest, annoy, inspire, or frighten us—are all the result of evolution. They are a response to something in our environment. Music evolved before language, and its responses stimulate many more areas in the brain than simple language. But why does it continue to exist?

"Purely for pleasure?" Dr. Susan Pauker postulates. "Many species sing: birds, whales, even dogs howling. Is that music? Is that art? Who can say? For humans, I think music is an extension of communication that gives pleasure. It stimulates endorphins and it stimulates serotonin uptake prevention and therefore makes people feel good.

"I adopted two puppies, and the first time I practiced music in front of them, they howled right along with me. I was laughing so hard, I could barely play. Over time they stopped, but I can't help wondering, What was that? Were they communicating with my music? Were they irritated? Was their 'wolfness' coming out in them?

"I was once on a roof with a friend in Santa Fe and we were listening to the coyotes. They are all communicating by these amazing high-pitched sounds all through the hills. Is that music? I think we don't understand how much music there is.

"Look at babies: very soon after they make good eye contact, they start making little sounds. Is that music to them? I don't know. When I am trying to figure out a child's developmental level, I start by singing 'Row Row Row Your Boat' or 'Twinkle Twinkle Little Star' or 'ABC.' I observe how well they are engaged. Music is part of my neurologic exam."

"The Greatest Thing in the World"

The Mexican-born Dr. Samuel Zyman is Professor of Music Theory at The Juilliard School in New York. His works are known for their intricate tonalities, fascinating rhythms that hint at his Latin origins, and, above all, their deep sense of humanity. I first heard Zyman's work in Caracas, when cellists Yo-Yo Ma and Carlos Prieto performed his *Suite for Two Cellos* for five hundred young cellists from Venezuela's *El Sistema* program. The two had commissioned Zyman to write "Suite for Two Cellos" for the reunion of their sister Stradivari instruments.

Dr. Zyman earned his M.D. from the University of Mexico but never practiced medicine, instead deciding to embrace a musical career. But he told me that he maintains his awareness of the connection between medicine and music. In an interview with *Juilliard Journal*, Zyman explained that "There was simply no comparison between the beauty and emotional power of music and such things as pathology, infectious diseases, or internal medicine (with all due respect to the medical profession)."[21]

"There is no question that there are physiological things in music—the heart is one of the most important ones. And breathing. In my music theory classes, sometimes I bring up a topic about medicine . . . for example, how the heart beats—anything from potassium pumps to the conduction system to the sinus atrial node and how it affects the heart. I sometimes mention the physiology of the heart when I'm talking about Stravinsky, for example. There are some passages in *The Rite of Spring* when there is a huge surge of energy that runs through the entire score, vertically. So I tell them this is a little like an electric discharge that you take from an electric machine—a defibrillator—and you apply it. It is a little like what you do when you want to destroy the rhythm of the heart in someone who is dying—you put the electrodes on and you reset the whole thing . . . it is that same sort of reset of rhythm in the Stravinsky."

Zyman said that his medical background even finds its way into his compositions. "Music is far and away the most powerful way for a human being to express himself. Music to me is the greatest thing in the world. And being a composer makes it safe to say what you want to say. There were some really shocking things that I saw when I was a medical student. There is nothing more painful than seeing kids who are suffering, or kids who have some terminal disease, such as cancer or kidney disease. I recall when we were rotating through the pediatric department and we would come to the hospital every day and become friends with the kids. But you never knew the next day if they were still going to be there, and there were so few resources."

As a pediatrician, I fully understand the medical experience he describes. Working with children is filled with the greatest joys—and most profound sorrows. As a musician, I can hear how Dr. Zyman has been able to express his experiences through the language of music in his unique compositions.

"Something Extra"

I've written earlier about Dr. Albert Schweitzer and what he refers to as the "fellowship of those who bear the mark of pain." A doctor who has experienced personal tragedy is more empathic toward her patients. An artist who has survived the Holocaust incorporates images of loss and disillusion in even the most beautiful of his paintings. And a violinist who has experienced trauma expresses his life's experiences through his primary language of music.

In the spring of 2006, conductor Jonathan McPhee called to tell me about a brilliant young violinist, Augustin Hadelich, who he wanted to engage for the following concert season. "He is a wonderful musician—beautiful tone, great technique and that *something extra* in his playing. Although he's only twenty-one and still a student at Juilliard, he already has a maturity of sound far beyond his years."

Indeed, Augustin Hadelich, in his twenty-one years, had already traveled a journey few will experience in a lifetime.

Raised on a farm in Tuscany, Hadelich's talent was discovered at an early age, and he was concertizing in Italy by the age of seven. He loved the violin and he had a rare, natural talent. But in 1999, when he was fifteen years old, Hadelich sustained severe burns to his face, upper chest and arms in a fire at his family home. Fortunately, his left hand was spared. But his right arm, the arm used to bow the violin, was contractured (a permanent shrinkage of a muscle or tendon) by scars. It took months of painful physical therapy to regain full extension of his arm.

"The doctors told me I would never play the violin again," Augustin told me a few years ago. "But they did not realize what that would mean to me and to my life."

As a pediatrician, I understand how much self-awareness and independence play a part in the development of a healthy adolescent. I can only imagine what young Augustin, who identified himself as a violinist, must have gone through at that time. "How could I not play? Hearing them say that made me so angry. I simply worked even harder to get better and to get back to playing."

Although his face and arms still bear the scars of his burns, Augustin Hadelich did not *just* get back to playing, he excelled. Only a few years after his accident, Hadelich graduated *summa cum laude* from Instituto Mascagni in Livorno, Italy, then enrolled at the prestigious Juilliard School in New York, pursuing its top degree, the prestigious Artist Diploma.

In an interview in the *New York Times*, Hadelich's Juilliard violin teacher, Joel Smirnoff, recalled, "His transition to thinking of himself as a child to adult was bound up with his transition from burn victim to normality again. Because he had to seriously work on that internally, I think it facilitated someone who showed up at Juilliard at age twenty with real maturity."

Thus we were thrilled to hear from his manager that Augustin Hadelich, a rising star, would be available to perform the Glazunov Violin Concerto with us in the final concert of the season in April 2007. By coincidence—or perhaps by karmic resonance—the Community Partner already scheduled for that April concert was the Shriners Hospital for Children, one of the top pediatric burn centers anywhere.

I had a long conversation with the young but insightful and wise Augustin Hadelich. Yes, he would be delighted to perform the Glazunov Violin Concerto with the Longwood Symphony. No, he had not realized that each of our concerts were collaborations with charities, but that was cool. And yes, he was comfortable that the concert was to benefit Shriners Burns Hospital. And finally . . . he hesitated . . . yes, he *would* be interested in visiting the children at the hospital to play for them.

On the day he visited Shriners Hospital, accompanied by some LSO members, Augustin was visibly nervous. It was the first time he had returned to a hospital since his accident and the memories were still so fresh. We were met by Dr. Robert Sheridan, the surgical director of the hospital. Dr. Sheridan, a surgeon by training and humanitarian by nature, explained that many of the children in the hospital were flown in for care they could not get in their home countries, separated from their families for long periods of time. Many required multi-staged corrective surgeries and returned repeatedly over many years.

I will never forget the flash of recognition in the eyes of those children when Augustin entered the room where the children, in wheelchairs and beds, were assembled. *The fellowship of those who bear the mark of pain.* Without a word, he took out his violin and simply played Bach.

Afterward, Augustin took questions from the children. When did you start the violin? What songs do you like? Then, a powerful question from the quiet young teenage girl covered in bandages, whose hospital bed had been wheeled into the room. She looked at him earnestly and said, in her native Spanish, "How did *you* do it? How did *you* leave here? What did you think about to get better?"

Augustin looked directly at her and answered her, also in Spanish: "Imagine yourself already out of here. Think of what you want to be doing *after* your time here, and aim to go *there.*" The young girl did not answer, but I could see from the glow in her eyes that she understood.

Brain Circuits

Those of us who see the healing power of music sometimes wonder: Will research someday advance to the point where specific pieces of music will be used to treat specific illnesses? In other words, will we ever write prescriptions for Bach or Haydn the way we now write for amoxicillin or Ambien?

"Perhaps," said Dr. Michael Barnett, the oboist. "I think that certainly in rehabilitation that time will come. And for doctors to recommend that people to engage either in producing or listening to different kinds of music will certainly happen, especially as a kind of adjunct to other rehabilitation. One of the great things we've learned in our symposia on music and the brain is that music really has an incredibly profound influence and involvement in multiple brain areas and circuits that are completely parallel to other processes we use in our daily life, like the way we speak and the way we act. There's something very powerful about having a way of expressing oneself in a completely parallel way to what we view as our normal mode. In rehab when we're trying to teach brain-injured people how to speak again, they may have trouble getting out even a single word. But if they can express themselves through music, that can be a way for them to regain access to damaged areas that have prevented them from speaking or behaving normally."

Barnett said he's seen a similar rewiring or detouring in the brains of patients suffering from Alzheimer's or other age-related diseases. "A lot of our elderly patients who get delirious in the hospital setting often respond to relaxing classical music that drowns out the beeps and drones and hustle-bustle of the hospital. I've definitely seen patients who seem to be a little more grounded when there is some music going on."

And they may even recognize/"become clear" mentally when a specific song comes on that they love, giving them a chance to escape the dementia for a short while. We'll see examples of this in Chapter Eleven.

An Adjunct Treatment

Dr. Daniela Krause is a flutist and piccolo player in the LSO. As a clinical pathologist at Massachusetts General Hospital whose specialty is transfusion medicine and leukemia research, she has devoted her career to caring for patients with cancer and seeking a cure. Born in Berlin, trained in Germany, the U.K., and the U.S., she speaks with a soft blend of English and German accents that reflect her dual heritage.

Dr. Krause speculates that the first mainstream doctors who might prescribe music as medicine would likely be psychologists and psychotherapists. "They might say to a patient, 'Look, instead of beating your head against the wall, why don't you go to a concert, enjoy some music and purge your emotion that way.'" She added thoughtfully, "I am too much of a medically trained person to say that we can cure cancer with music, just like we can't cure cancer with just herbs. But I think that as an adjunct therapy to cancer treatment—or as adjunct therapy to almost any kind of treatment, really—music is the way to go.

"When I was a medical student at the Eden Marie Curie Cancer Care hospice in London I observed the different things that people choose to do during their last days of life. Some people go through their stamp collection for the last time. Some people sit in the garden looking at the daffodils. But often, people want to hear their favorite music once more. It may be Beethoven or an opera or a folk song that has personal meaning and is connected to very specific memories. It's really a very individualized thing. It's important for patients to have the choice of different styles of music, whichever helps. Patients often turn to music as the final medicine in the moment when their illness is about to overtake them. They know something about music that we doctors should pay attention to. If music can help doctors rethink their therapy with regards to something that will specifically help their specific patient, then I think we are on the right path. It is like 'personalized medicine' from a different angle. Instead of sequencing the genetic information of a tumor, we are listening to what kind of music means the most and has the most positive impact on a patient."

7

Music and Brain Development

SUSPENDED IN AMNIOTIC FLUID IN the darkness of the womb, where taste, smell, touch, and sight are all deadened, the first thing a human senses of the outside world comes through the ears: the steady rhythm of its mother's heart. We know a baby hears, because it can be jolted by a sharp sound like a slamming door or a popping balloon. A baby can already recognize its mother's voice—and her songs—even before it's born.

But it all starts with the primal rhythm of the heartbeat that gave you life in there. That rhythm stays with us through all our adult experience with music.

The first piece of music is already in place before birth.

As a pediatrician, I get a glimpse of the future in the children I treat. So many of our psychological challenges have their roots in this formative time—but so do our lifelong interests, our hobbies, and, yes, our spirits. Nearly all my LSO colleagues were introduced to music, to medicine, or both, when they were children, as we saw in the last chapter. But music affects us all from a very early age, whether or not we are consciously aware of it.

Doctor of pediatric surgery and violinist Terry Buchmiller knows how children develop. With chestnut hair that she keeps in a ponytail and intense eyes, she sparkles with energy, often snapping her fingers as she speaks. She is a marathoner and definitely has a runner's physique. Her soft voice belies the incredible strength within—she is one of the few females in her field of surgery (the American College of Surgeons has eighteen thousand members, only twenty-five percent of whom are women). Her field is even more rarified: Terry specializes in fetal surgery—surgery on the unborn child in order to try to correct life-threatening congenital anomalies before the baby is born.

She approaches music as she does surgery—with a methodical, cool determination, a laser focus and unwavering quest for excellence. She has served as concertmistress of the orchestra on occasion. In March 2011, we performed the Boston premiere of a work by David Kechley (Williams College) which contained some very tough violin solos for the concertmaster. Terry worked with the composer, sought out advice from violin professionals (including my husband), and was able to borrow a beautiful old Italian instrument for the concert performance (untouchable in price even for a pediatric surgeon). She received rave reviews from the audience and the composer, who was in the audience that night.

It was a pediatrician who introduced her to medicine when she was just nine years old, about the same time that she began to play the violin. Buchmiller's favorite toy was "Operation," in which you had to use a pair of tweezers to carefully remove body parts with funny names ("wish bone," "broken heart," "spare rib") without setting off a buzzer. She was full of questions for her own doctor who asked if she wanted to sit with him in the office and see patients.

"Those were very different days. I can't imagine having a nine-year-old follow me around in my practice now. But he even let me watch an endoscopic procedure. I later saw surgery at age eleven in the UCSF operating theatre. That was it! I loved it! It was absolutely fascinating."

Her interest in medicine grew apace with her music. She worked as a candy-striper when she was fifteen and volunteered in the emergency room "because that's where all the exciting stuff happened." When she went to college, she majored in music, but "I always knew I was going to be premed." Her guidance counselor and other adult advisors were concerned. It looked like she was being pulled in two directions. But there was no conflict to Buchmiller. She believes the two pastimes have overlapping skill sets.

"What makes you a great musician?" she asked. "You have to break things down, repeat them, practice them over and over and over again, and then take a step back and put the emotional and mental pieces together to make it into a whole. It's the same with being a great surgeon. There are many little pieces, many tiny skills that you knit together in ever-changing ways. You practice them over and over and over and over again until you get them perfect. Think about suturing. You're tying the same tiny knot over and over and every one has to be perfect because someone's life is on the line. You're saving a life one tiny knot at a time.

"I remember one of my teachers at the San Francisco Conservatory saying all we were going to do the following week was the eight bars of the opening of the Mendelssohn Violin Concerto. The teacher said, 'All I want you to do for five hours a day is practice the opening eight bars.' So I played those eight bars a thousand different ways until I found the one way I thought Mendelssohn wanted it to be expressed. That kind of repetition, experimentation and exploration ingrained not only a skill, but a whole pattern of thought, a whole structure for approaching the world."

In a 2007 article in the Harvard Business Review, Professor K. Anders Ericsson wrote: "The journey to truly superior performance is neither for the faint of heart nor for the impatient. The development of genuine expertise requires struggle, sacrifice, and honest, often painful self-assessment. There are no shortcuts. It will take you at least a decade to achieve expertise, and you will need to invest that time wisely, by engaging in 'deliberate' practice—practice that focuses on tasks beyond your current level of competence and comfort." Professor Ericsson went on to describe his research that it takes ten thousand hours of practice to achieve expert level at any skill, a point that became the central theme of Malcolm Gladwell's successful book on success, *The Outliers: The Story of Success*.[1, 2]

Dr. Buchmiller continues: "Playing music teaches you to break a big task down into smaller tasks so you can master the skills of each. When you put these small pieces together, it creates the whole. It's the same if you are performing an operation. You must master each separate tiny skill so that when you put them together, you have mastered the form and function of the entire procedure. And you have to have enough experience so that you can deal with the nuances as they arise. It's not that a great performer in music never makes a mistake. It's just that they adjust for it so quickly that the rest of the world doesn't notice, so it still sounds perfect. The same thing happens during an operation. Everything cannot be perfectly under your control at all times, but you make an adjustment so seamlessly and so quickly that in the end it turns out to be that 'perfect operation.'

"There's a special dedication to being a great musician or a great doctor, You don't just happen on it. You lock yourself up in a practice room for hours and hours and hours. And you really focus and you do repetitive tasks and then you back off from that and then you let that whole connection happen. That process is so intertwined with both professions that, in a way, they are not different skills at all."

Neuroplasticity

Does playing music actually foster better cognitive thinking in the developing minds of all children—or is the ability to play music one of the distinguishing marks of an intelligent child? It's the classic question: nurture or nature?

A 2010 study[3] by researchers at Northwestern University found that "active engagement with musical sounds enhances neuroplasticity"—defined as "the ability of the brain to adapt and change to new experience—and 'enables the nervous system to provide the stable scaffolding of meaningful patterns so important to learning.'" The study found that children who are musically trained developed better reading ability and a better vocabulary overall than children who weren't musically trained.

In their 2009 study "Musical Training Shapes Structural Brain Development," researchers Krisa L. Hyde, Jason Lerch, and their colleagues explored the "nature vs. nurture" question about whether musicians' brains are naturally specially adapted to playing music, or if their playing music from an early age somehow altered the way their brains work. Their findings came down heavily on the side of the latter: "We demonstrate[d] structural brain changes after only fifteen months of musical training in early childhood, which were correlated with improvements in musically relevant motor and auditory skills," they wrote. "These findings shed light on brain plasticity and suggest that structural brain differences in adult experts (whether musicians or experts in other areas) are likely due to training-induced brain plasticity."[4]

In the early 1990s, *Nature* magazine published a widely discussed paper purporting to show that listening to Mozart's piano sonata K 448 in D major improves children's IQ by nine or ten points. That quickly led to a whole industry that packaged classical music for babies—even pre-natal babies—including "Baby Mozart" and other similar CDs and dot-coms.

The practice got a black eye in 2009 when the Federal Trade Commission found that the popular "Baby Einstein" line of recordings and toys had no power to increase brainpower, as the packaging seemed to imply. The cornerstone of these products was classical music, notably Mozart. The $200 million Disney-owned company (whose DVDs included "Baby Mozart," "Baby Shakespeare," and "Baby Galileo") was ordered to offer refunds for up to four of the products per household sold since 2004.

A *New York Times* article on the issue quoted a letter from a group of public health lawyers who had threatened a class-action suit: "The Walt Disney Company's entire Baby Einstein marketing regime is based on express and implied claims that their videos are educational and beneficial for early childhood development." The letter branded the claims "false because research shows that television viewing is potentially harmful for very young children." [5]

Their claims may have been inflated, but I still believe in the importance of exposure to music at a young age, Baby Einstein or not. Significantly, the focus of objection was on the video element, not the musical element of the claims.

On this issue the hard research is mixed, partly because it remains a difficult thing to measure. "On brain development there have been a few studies that have said that classical music can help," Dr. Buchmiller said, "especially with newborns who are so sick that they cannot be held, cannot even be touched, so they are not getting the audiological cues that they would have at home being nursed with their families. Research has shown that all those cues help promote brain development. Music is the one thing that can help with those babies, and anything that promotes that environment is a healing environment."

Whether or not a baby is ill, music (not video) has indeed been found to have a positive effect. "The babies find the music very calming," Dr. Buchmiller said. "We've found in our Neo-natal Intensive Care Unit that if classical music is played versus not, the babies actually gain weight quicker. So it has a physiological effect as well."

Some parents believe that playing classical music is good for very young babies, and I agree. At every instant, the baby is growing and learning. The language of touch, taste, and sound are all new to them and they respond to every stimuli. If exposed, the baby learns the unique pattern of music as easily as the patterns of speech. Some parents even play music for their children when they are still in utero, on the theory that there is something in the music that will stimulate fetal brain development. While I don't discourage this, the sight of pregnant women with headphones on their bellies or an earbud in their navel seems a little extreme! But why not? We know that babies can hear ambient sound. Why not music— soft, ambient music—as well?

"Having said that, exposing your baby to different stimuli when in the womb isn't a bad thing by any means," the magazine said. "If you do choose to directly expose your baby to music in utero, either by stretching headphones over your tummy or by holding a radio at stomach level, you should limit this to gentle music, played at a low level, for a maximum of one hour a day to avoid overstimulating your unborn baby.

"If you would like to expose your baby to music in the womb but would prefer not to take such direct measures then don't worry, your baby will be able to hear any music that you do (as amnotic fluid is a good conductor of sound waves). Having a radio playing as you go about your day or sitting with your feet up and listening to your favorite CD, will sufficiently expose your baby to the rhythm of the music."

MUSIC AND IQ

We now come back to our friend Dr. Psyche Loui, the LSO violinist and neurology researcher. In January 2011, Dr. Loui led a team of LSO members to host the second of our symposia "Crossing the Corpus Callosum: Neuroscience, Healing and Music."

"Does listening to one piano sonata for ten minutes or so *really* improve your IQ? It turns out that's pretty much dead," Dr. Loui said. "But nevertheless, there is lots of evidence that long-term engagement in making music and listening to music does impact your brain in many positive ways. For instance, we found that people who practice musical instruments for more than two hours a week have larger corpus callosums, which is the brain area that connects the left and right brains. So there's bigger connectivity, more efficient connectivity, between left hemisphere and right hemisphere of the brain in people who practice more. It's also been shown that conductors in general have larger corpus callosums, which makes sense because you need to be really good at homing in on exactly which instrument among seventy is a bit out of tune. That kind of accuracy requires a lot of brain connectivity."

In a *Nature Reviews* magazine piece, "The Musician's Brain as a Model of Neuroplasticity," Thomas F. Münte, Eckart Altenmüller, and Lutz Jäncke surveyed a tidal wave of evidence that playing music not only stimulates the brain, but actually rewires it and stimulates changes and growth in areas "that are involved in motor and auditory processing." They wrote, "Interestingly, musicians who began their musical training before the age of seven have a larger anterior midsagittal corpus callosum than controls or musicians who started training later. Because the size of the midsagittal corpus callosum is a good indicator of the number of axons that cross the midline, this finding indicates that this subgroup of musicians has an enhanced interaction between the two hemispheres. This hypothesis has been corroborated by a bilateral transcranial magnetic stimulation (TMS) study in pianists and guitarists, which revealed decreased interhemispheric inhibition. This, in turn, might facilitate bimanual coordination in musicians by increasing signal transfer between the hemispheres. . . . Male musicians [the group that was studied] have been shown to have a greater mean relative cerebellar volume than male non-musicians."[6, 7]

What does all that mean? It might not be as simple as the upward tick of IQ points (and IQ measurements are misleading anyway), but the positive influence of music on the brain can now be measured. In musician's brains, not only are the connections between the two sides of the brain increased, but the volume of the brain itself is increased. And the younger one starts music, the better.

EARLY MEMORIES

Children have the ability to recognize melodies from a very early age. In fact, the singing tradition was a way to pass on knowledge from generation to generation, even before written language was developed. Nursery rhymes, for example, have been passed on through the centuries. Not only an appealing way to communicate with preschoolers, these songs are also educational: teaching them cautionary tale such as "Jack and Jill," or helping them with rote memory such as "The Alphabet Song."

Engagement with music starts young. In her book The Power of Music: Pioneering Discoveries in the New Science of Song, Elena Mannes reported on a study by Sandra Trehub of the University of Toronto, in which Trehub exposed babies to patterns of notes that were either consonant or dissonant, in order to see, first, if they could tell the difference between the two, and, second, if they preferred one over the other, based on the perceived reactions of the babies. The tests showed that "babies could detect very tiny differences" between consonant and dissonant patterns, and that "if the babies had a choice, they spent more time listening to the consonant music," though subsequent research found that the preference "may be at least somewhat due to learning."[8] Music tapped into something very deep inside the minds of these children, and it impressed its effects very early in life.

While I believe that all children are born with innate musical sensibility, some young people are born with a particular talent in music. One of my neighbors, a cellist and neurologist, related a story about their colicky four-month old son. At wits' end, he and his wife pulled out a CD of music by Vivaldi. Much to their surprise, the baby began to laugh. When they turned it off he started screaming again. So they turned it back on and he started laughing again. I saw him a few years ago when he was freshman at Harvard and said "You know your Dad keeps telling me this story about how he played The Four Seasons for you. What was so funny?" And he said, "It wasn't *The Four Seasons*. There's nothing funny about *The Four Seasons*. Don't you know? It was a Vivaldi violin concerto." It must have been a Bach violin concerto. Now that's funny!

Right and Wrong Music for Kids?

Parents also ask me if there is one kind of music that is better than another for their children after they are born. The Baby Einstein people will tell you that classical is best, and I would actually tend to agree, because I believe it is the most complex and satisfying, and engages the brain in a unique way. But I know parents who prefer rock music and want their children to be exposed as early as possible, and parents who feel the same about Broadway music, country music, various ethnic musics, even church music (for those who believe the development of the soul is as important as that of the brain). In the end, it is something that reflects the parents' interests more than the child's. It is part of a parent's job to expose their children to culture they believe will help the child develop as a citizen of their world. And children's minds are like sponges. They will absorb video-game music and advertising jingles as readily as anything else.

I would say that *any* music that is not annoying or upsetting to the child and that has appropriate lyrics (as determined by the parent) is good for the child. But keep in mind that whatever music you choose, "children will listen," as Stephen Sondheim wrote in *Into the Woods*. I can still remember the lullabies my mother sang to me when I was a child, just as Christopher did his Vivaldi.

They may be among my earliest identifiable memories. I still remember jump-rope and other playground chants I learned before I began school. Music sticks with a child and helps form an important part of the matrix of her or his development.

MUSIC AND AUTISM

Music therapy has been employed in a variety of settings and used to help a variety of mental and physical challenges. But some of the most significant work in recent years has been devoted to using music to treat children suffering with autism, which is characterized by varying degrees of disengagement from the normal concerns and interactions of life. Diagnoses of autism have been rising steadily for the past two decades, and when parents come into my office their concern verges at times on panic. Researchers are still trying to determine the precise cause of autism, while doctors are working hard to find treatments, if not yet cures. It seems that music, in addition to Applied Behavior Analysis (ABA) is one of the most effective treatments—listening to it and, especially, playing it. Lots of studies agree.

In a March 2008 survey of the research, the American Music Therapy Association found "Music therapy is a particularly important intervention for children with autism spectrum disorders to engage and foster their capacity for flexibility, creativity, variability, and tolerance of change, in order to balance the more structured and behaviorally driven education required in school settings. . . . Research supports connections between speech and singing, rhythm and motor behavior, memory for song and memory for academic material, and overall ability of preferred music to enhance mood, attention, and behavior to optimize the student's ability to learn and interact."[9]

In children with autism, music can have an even more profound effect.

Dr. Juliette Alvin in her groundbreaking 1978 book *Music Therapy for the Autistic Child* (updated in 1992 with Auriel Warwick) gave detailed descriptions of the author's own research into the different ways autistic children responded to music.[10] Even those children who might not develop meaningful speech demonstrated a proclivity to music.

Dr. Myra J. Staum, Director and Professor of Music Therapy at Willamette University in Salem, Oregon, wrote "It has been noted time and again that autistic children evidence unusual sensitivities to music. Some have perfect pitch, while many have been noted to play instruments with exceptional musicality. Music therapists traditionally work with autistic children because of this unusual responsiveness which is adaptable to non-music goals Some children have unusual sensitivities only to certain sounds. One boy, after playing a xylophone bar, would spontaneously sing up the harmonic series from the fundamental pitch. Through careful structuring, syllable sounds were paired with his singing of the harmonics and the boy began incorporating consonant-vowel sounds into his vocal play. Soon simple 2-3 note tunes were played on the xylophone by the therapist who modeled more complex verbalizations, and the child gradually began imitating them."

More recently, in the April 2010 *Journal of Music Therapy*, Dr. Hayoung A. Lim documented the impact of music in teaching autistic children to speak. She observed that "Children with ASD perceive important linguistic information embedded in music stimuli organized by principles of pattern perception, and produce the functional speech."

DR. STAUM ALSO USES MUSIC to help children learn to interact socially. "Musical games like passing a ball back and forth to music or playing sticks and cymbals with another person might be used to foster this interaction. Eye contact might be encouraged with imitative clapping games near the eyes or with activities which focus attention on an instrument played near the face. Preferred music may be used contingently for a wide variety of cooperative social behaviors like sitting in a chair or staying with a group of other children in a circle."

She described how simple chants could be used to impart social lessons while stimulating language development. "One six-year-old echolalic child was taught speech by having the therapist/teacher sing simple question/answer phrases set to a familiar melody with full rhythmic and harmonic accompaniment The child held the objects while singing:

"Do you eat an apple? Yes, yes.
Do you eat an apple? Yes, yes.
Do you eat an apple? Yes, yes.
Yes, yes, yes.

"and

"Do you eat a pencil? No, no.

Do you eat a pencil? No, no.
Do you eat a pencil? No, no.
No, no, no." [11]

Finally, in a meta-analysis of nine different studies on the subject published in the *Journal of Music Therapy*, Jennifer Whipple weighed the studies in terms of how many people were studied, the various ages of the subjects, how rigorous the researchers were, how music was selected, and how it was exposed to the study subjects. She concluded that "all music intervention, regardless of purpose or implementation, has been effective for children and adolescents with autism." [12]

"ABSOLUTELY FASCINATING"

I've described how Dr. Buchmiller discovered her interest in music and medicine when she was about nine. Dr. Psyche Loui started even earlier, at age five, with piano lessons, and switched to violin when she was seven. She credits her parents with her ability to stick with a problem. "There were definitely points at which I had a little attention deficit when I was little, and I wanted to play or watch TV instead of practice. It was my parents who insisted, 'No, you're going to stick to the practicing,' and I thank them for that many years down the road.

"When I went to college at Duke University in North Carolina I started taking psychology courses. There were many great professors who taught me a lot and were very encouraging, like Jonathan Bagg of the Ciompi Quartet. At Duke I started looking at musical scores and wanting to study psychology and music together. I was a psychology and music double major and ended up doing two theses. I analyzed Leonard Bernstein's *Serenade after Plato's Symposium*, which is a violin concerto essentially, but is modeled after Plato's Symposium. I also read Bernstein's Norton Lectures, in which he tries to answer the big question 'whither music?'—where does music come from, where should it go? It uses linguistic principles to analyze elements of music. For my senior thesis I performed the *Serenade* and wrote a paper about how Bernstein applied the theoretical principles to his composition.

"And in Psychology, I got very interested in my current line of work, looking at brain responses to musical chords and chord progressions. I did my senior thesis on the effects of attention on how the brain processes Western musical chord progressions. So if you hear a C major piece, it should end in C major, but if it doesn't end in C major, you can record these brain potentials that say 'Oh, that is really surprising.' There's a classic brain response for that. And we looked at how that brain response changes as a function of whether you're paying attention to the music you're listening to or whether you're just doing some reading with music in the background. And it turns out that paying attention does enhance these brain potentials, as you would predict. So that was the senior thesis, and I was just absolutely hooked. It was absolutely fascinating."

"EL SISTEMA"

I have had a chance to see the question of nature versus nurture in child development illustrated vividly starting in 2001 when I became fascinated with a Venezuelan organization whose full name is *Fundación del Estado para el Sistema Nacional de las Orquestas Juveniles e Infantiles de Venezuela* ("National Network of Youth and Children's Orchestras of Venezuela"), but commonly called just *El Sistema* ("The System").

El Sistema was founded in 1975 by Maestro Jose Antonio Abreu, a musician, economist, and politician, who had a vision that poor children and children at risk of falling into lives of crime or drug abuse could find a new life through music. Since that time, more than a quarter of a million Venezuelan children have participated in some one hundred and twenty-five youth orchestras around that nation, and the program and its philosophy are being exported to other countries, including, in a nascent form, the U.S.

Maestro Abreu says the program was not meant to create musicians but to create socially engaged young citizens who learn *Tocar y Lucar,* to "Play and Fight" (work out their competitive urges), in the socially safe environment of music. Together, the children struggle up against Mahler, and they can "fight" with each other about a phrase or about playing in tune. Together, they work until they get it right. They keep moving forward, pursuing what Maestro Abreu terms "an affluence of spirit." They forge new bonds and learn to communicate. And no one gets hurt. It is an intense after-school music program, but the students also learn about community and collaboration, and teach each other. When they graduate, they are encouraged to pursue other fields, and many do. While there, I found many musicians interested in going into medicine, dentistry, and engineering. Now that the program is thirty-five years old, we are beginning to see evidence of an entirely new generation of musical physicians there.

Interestingly, all of us in the Longwood Symphony had a chance to experience some of that wonderful Venezuelan discipline mixed with a pure love of the music, through our conductor Maestro Francisco Noya, as mentioned earlier. Born in Caracas and a contemporary of Maestro Abreu, he became an accomplished cellist and conductor there before moving to the United States to study at Boston University. A man with a generous soul, infectious laugh, and "affluence of spirit," he helped the LSO thrive through the years that we developed our community programs.

When I first encountered *El Sistema* for myself in Caracas, I was serving as a pediatrician chaperone for a tour to Venezuela with the Youth Philharmonic Orchestra at the New England Conservatory, one of the U.S.'s top high school youth orchestras in the country. The YPO is conducted by visionary musician Benjamin Zander, and the Preparatory Division of NEC was led by Mark Churchill, who served as its dean for thirty years. Both men are passionate about the importance of music in the lives of young people, and thousands of children throughout New England have benefited from this passion.

My daughter, a high school sophomore and violinist, was gracious enough to allow her mother to join her on our adventure to Venezuela. We arrived in Caracas expecting to be playing with modestly talented kids from a developing country. What we found was a immense ensemble of two hundred and fifty talented young people who were as good as or better than our kids—a shock to our students with their American sensibility who had believed that they were the best in the world. Here were fabulous young musicians, some as young as nine years old, who were serious and passionate about their music, enthusiastic about meeting other musicians like themselves, and completely open to learning and sharing. Within a few days, the American and Venezuelan kids had totally fallen love with each other and any barrier, including language, had given way to their mutual excitement about music. Soon there were groups of students in every corner of the schoolyard—young violinists playing the difficult Mendelssohn Violin Concerto together in one corner and percussionists sharing techniques on how to play Venezuelan *maracas* in the other corner—a bond had been forged between the U.S. system and the Venezuelan *El Sistema*. We capped our visit with four hundred kids playing on stage together, with American and Venezuelan musicians playing Tchaikovsky's *Romeo and Juliet Overture* together, sitting side by side.

I needed to learn more. I discovered that eighty percent of these kids were from homes below the Venezuelan poverty line, and many had witnessed domestic violence or had been victims of street violence or domestic violence themselves.

Maestro Abreu said his goal is to give children, through music, a reason to live and a reason to rise above the circumstances in which they live. To raise their sights he chose classical music at the highest level possible. He handed them good music and good instruments and challenged them to meet the highest standards. To get funding, Abreu cannily wrote *El Sistema* into the government budget as a social program rather than as an arts and culture program, which is what has allowed it to survive four administrations, including that of

President Hugo Chavez, who has actually been the hardest one to live with, of course. But it's still surviving, and has acquired an international reputation. It has been described by international leaders, such as Sir Simon Rattle, conductor of the Berlin Philharmonic, as "the future of classical music." If the program were to go down, there would rightfully be international condemnation now.

I've been fortunate to have gone back to Venezuela four times since then. Each time was a critical moment of change in the relationship of *El Sistema* with the United States. In 2001, NEC's Youth Philharmonic Orchestra performed with the Venezuelan Youth Orchestra to mark the founding of the Youth Orchestra of the Americas. The second time, again with the Youth Philharmonic Orchestra, a Friendship Agreement was signed between New England Conservatory and *El Sistema*. The third time is when my daughter Jennifer wrote her thesis on *El Sistema*, the first serious paper in English about the program. The fourth was with cellists Yo-Yo Ma and Carlos Prieto. The fifth was in summer 2010 when I traveled there with my husband and musical colleagues to teach chamber music to these top-level kids. The wonderful surprise was that ten years later, these students are now twenty-five years old and looking to see what they are going to do with their lives. The system created thousands upon thousands of musicians, and many of them told us that they are going to medical school! So many of the Venezuelan medical school applicants are *El Sistema* alumni that I wouldn't be surprised if, within a decade, seventy-five to one hundred percent of that nation's new doctors are graduates of this program. As a result, we may see LSOs popping up all over that country!

My experience with *El Sistema* has affected me deeply. At first I thought it was just part of my love for children and my love for education. Now I see something deeper. I see it as something positive for children to do that is not destroying each other and not destroying the world. *El Sistema* is creating a new generation of future leaders who have learned, through music, the true sense and value of community and collaboration. Whether they grow up to be doctors, bussiness people, or musicians, they understand *Tocar y Lucar.*

SHARPENING THE YOUNG BRAIN

As incredible as *El Sistema* is, there is no special magic in the way the Venezuelan kids respond to music. Music is innate in all children. As a pediatrician for twenty-five years, who deals with kids from birth up to age twenty-two, I can tell you that we're all wired for music from our earliest days. I have many patients who will "pitch-match"—which means that if you sing to them, they will sing back to you on the exact same pitch. Every time I weigh a child on my scale, which looks like a little boat, I sing "Row Row Row Your Boat." Most of them will vocalize in ways that match my pitch, even down to the age of eighteen months. A lot of babies like to be in the boat, and I think some of them would like to just sit in the scale forever and sing. When I give them their shots, I sing "Old MacDonald Had a Farm." They tend not to cry—or cry a little less—if they are engaged in listening to the song. Their pain centers are lessened because they are singing with me, looking in my eyes and trusting me. On a good day, it seems that rarely ten percent of my patients cry when they're getting shots, and I attribute that low number, not to my technique, but to our musical engagement through singing.

Sometimes I encounter children who have taught themselves to read by the age of three or four. Their parents come to me worried that the children might act out or become bored in kindergarten—and they probably will, to a certain extent. To those parents I say: time to start the piano. An instrument is a challenge that you can never fully conquer completely. There's always one more piece ahead of you, or there's always one more difficult thing that you can achieve. Or the piece that you have played for years can always be refined, retuned, or reinterpreted. That kind of challenge sharpens the brain.

One of my favorite patients was Ricky, who started the clarinet in his public elementary school. With encouragement, he thrived. Ricky came to my office at age eight for his annual appointment, clarinet in hand, and, to my delight, took it out and played "When the Saints Go Marching In!" He was a bright boy, perhaps not challenged enough in school, who found endless delight in working his way through pieces on his instrument. Doing that taught him lessons about patience, hard work, and self-discipline as valuable as any in the classroom. There was the added delight in the act of putting music out into the world, setting a room full of air vibrating with a bouncy march, and the reward of seeing the delight on the faces of his parents and doctor. Years later, as he graduated from my care, he brought me a CD of his band playing in New York's Carnegie Hall.

Unfortunately, that inborn love of music sometimes gets extinguished as the child grows older and finds other distractions like TV, team sports, the Internet, etc. I've seen parents deliberately try to stamp out interest in music in boys out of a fear that it will "waste" time that should be devoted to sports or other pursuits that they perceive as more practical. This generation of parents rarely encourages their children to engage in things that take a long time to accomplish. It may take years of playing music to get good enough to realize how much you like it. Parents sometimes make the mistake of asking the kids if they like to practice. If the kids say they don't, well, that's it. The parents let them stop. Imagine if the same policy were employed with homework! Professional musicians assure me that there were times when they were kids that they wanted to stay out to play for that extra thirty minutes rather than return to their instruments. Some even admit feeling the same way now. Like homework, I'd recommend letting the child stretch for a few minutes, smile sympathetically, and then say "That's fine, now let's keep practicing."

In the case of my own children, my son, who is now an accomplished violist, responded to the seeming magic that occurs with practice and discipline. If he was struggling with a particularly hard passage, I would sometimes encourage him to let it go until morning and assure him that his brain was continuing to learn it in his sleep. Very often, that *was* the case, and the musical phrase came easier in the morning.

These are the lucky kids—the ones who have had a chance to choose their music. So many don't even get the opportunity to play anymore because schools have cut back on arts education programs, and because of the expense of private lessons. Music is ubiquitous in society, but the gift of creating and playing an instrument, unfortunately, is not. For many, the next time kids encounter music, it's not as a musician or a singer. It's usually in a strictly passive form, listening to pop music in jingles on TV or on their iPods. Still, it's music, and every generation, as different as they may be from one another, has one thing in common. We've never had a generation yet that didn't hunger to listen to its own beat.

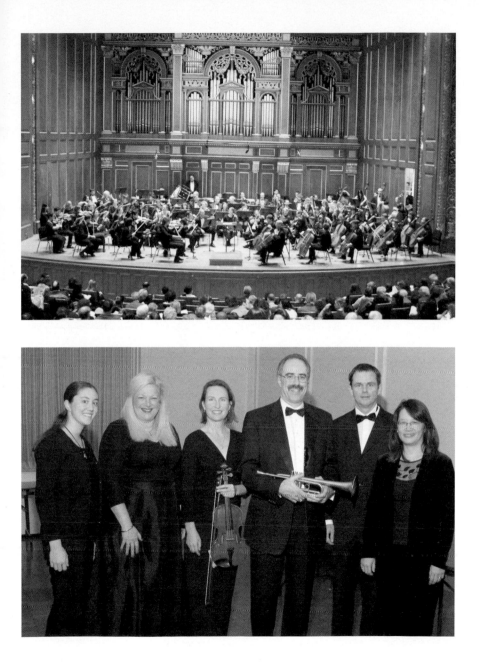

ABOVE: The Longwood Symphony Orchestra onstage at Jordan Hall. BELOW: Elisha Wachman, Sue Pauker, Heidi Harbison, Len Zon, Wolfram Goessling, and Lisa Wong before a concert. *Photos courtesy of the author.*

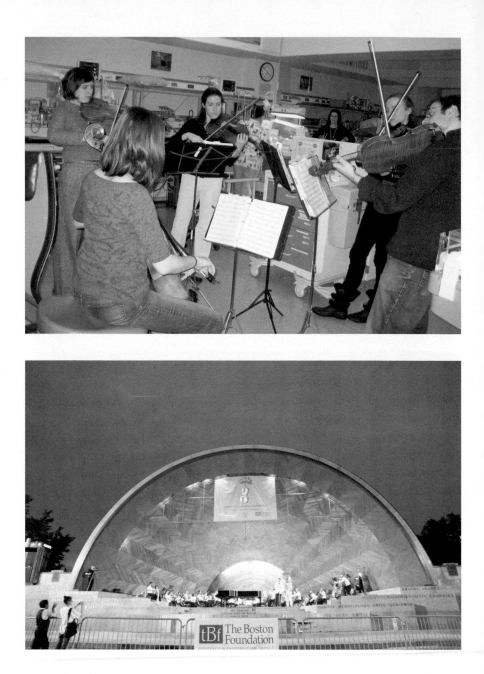

ABOVE: The "LSO on Call" in a Neonatal ICU. Young children, especially babies, are extremely sensitive to music. BELOW: The Longwood Symphony performs at the Hatch Memorial Shell on the *Esplandade* Boston. *Photos courtesy of the author.*

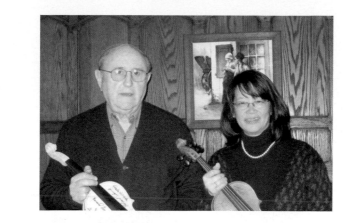

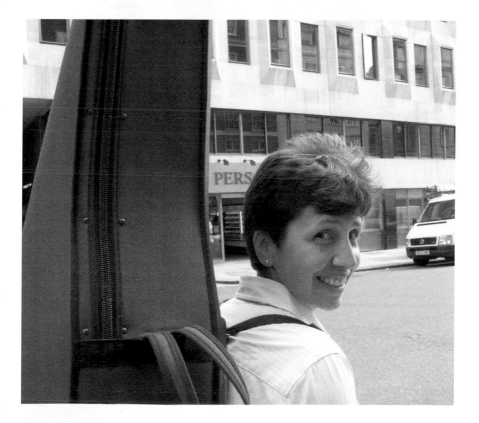

ABOVE: Bernard Lown and Lisa Wong with their violins. BELOW: Denise Lotufo in London on tour with the LSO. *Photos courtesy of the author.*

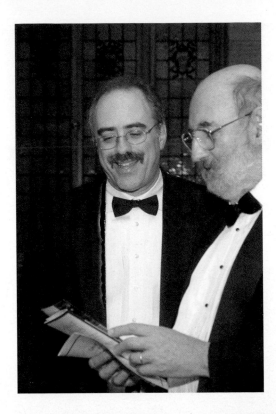

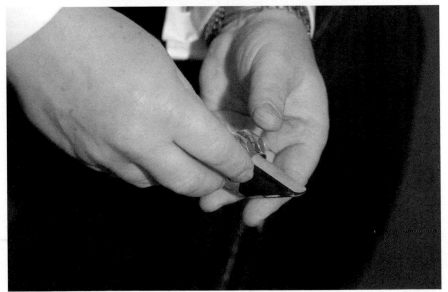

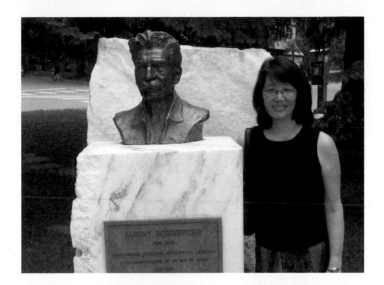

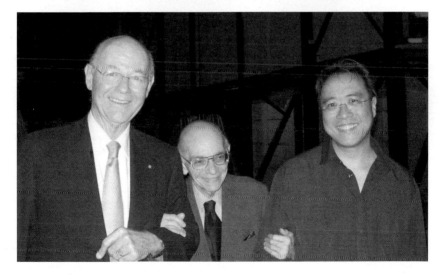

OPPOSITE ABOVE: Len Zons and Dr. Bill Kates before a concert. OPPOSITE BELOW: A clarinet reed. Like the oboe reed, a clarinet reed is extremely delicate and its vibrations are what create the clarinet's unique tone and sound. ABOVE: Lisa Wong in Aspen for the dedication and premier of the Albert Schweitzer memorial. Schweitzer's "Reverence for Life" philosophy and the integration of the humanities with science and medicine have profoundly influenced the LSO and other doctors and musicians around the world. BELOW: Cellists Carlos Prieto and Yo-Yo Ma with Jose Anonio Abreu in Venezuela. *Photos courtesy of the author.*

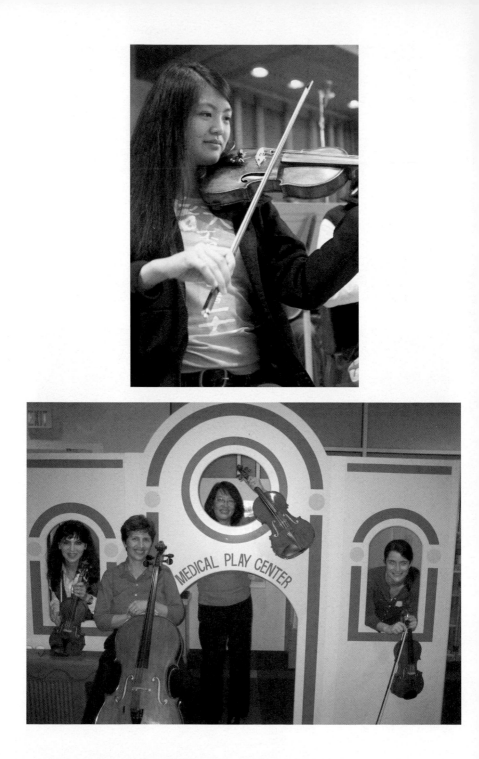

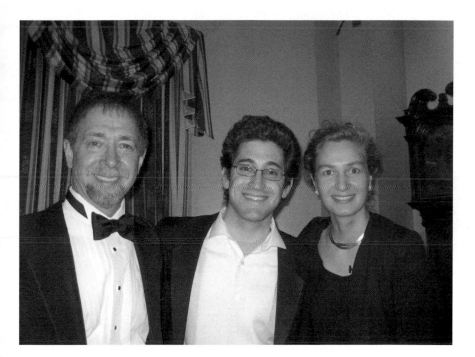

OPPOSITE ABOVE: LSO violinist Psyche Loui. OPPOSITE BELOW: The "LSO on Call" at the Shriners Hospital for Children's Burn Unit in Boston, where Augustine Hadelich also played for the burn victims. ABOVE: LSO members Tom Sheldon, Michael Barnett, and Daniela Krause. *Photos courtesy of the author.*

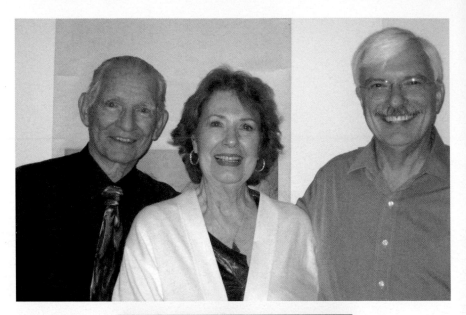

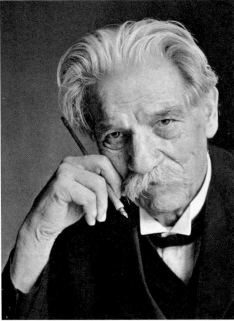

ABOVE: Longwood Symphony Orchestra founders Guy and Nalora Steele and Charles Kessler. *Photo courtesy of the author.* BELOW: Dr. Albert Schweitzer, the "patron saint" of the LSO and winner of the Nobel Peace Prize in 1952. *Photo courtesy of The Albert Schweitzer Fellowship®, www.schweitzerfellowship.org.*

Left and Right Hemispheres

To UNDERSTAND HOW MUSIC AFFECTS us, we need to understand, step by step, how the mind receives and processes music.

To start with, what is the brain made of? What makes up this most precious organ of our body? One of the earliest discoveries about the human brain—going back to the 1700 B.C. document known as the Edwin Smith Surgical Papyrus—is that it is actually not a single mass of nerve tissue, but divided into different sections, with different functions. The outer brain, known as the cerebrum or neocortex, is the convoluted "gray matter" where most of higher cognitive function, such as reasoning, language, and learning takes place. The mid-brain is the home of our pleasure centers and important for routing of information; and the medulla—the most ancient part of the brain, connected to the spine, controls our movement, breathing, and heartbeat.

The cortex, which is more highly developed in humans than in other species, is divided into two lobes or hemispheres, the left and the right, connected by a cable of nerve tissue called the corpus callosum. In a sense, we have two brains that work together. Each has slightly different jobs and processes different kinds of information in different ways. The left brain controls the right side of the body, and vice versa. The brain also hosts a variety of specialized bodies like the hypothalamus and the hippocampus, which help us form emotional responses.

All these are things we know. What researchers are discovering is how complex and fascinating the nerve pathways within the brain can be.

I thought of a musical experience that Dr. Daniela Krause and I shared not long ago. Dr. Krause, a German-born flutist, specializes in transfusion medicine and leukemia research. As part of LSO on Call, she recalled, "We took a quartet to a nursing home to play for Alzheimer's patients. Some of them hadn't spoken in months, or even years. We started with a Mozart flute quartet, which is jolly music. Then we picked out some show tunes from *My Fair Lady* and *Mary Poppins,* and suddenly these people who had not been able to talk or communicate were singing and clapping." All four of our musicians had personal connections to people in our families with dementia or Alzheimer's, and our performance was not only profoundly moving to the caregivers and nursing staff, but to the musicians as well.

"My father had Parkinson's disease with presenile dementia. He was completely confused all the time. But every time he got agitated or annoyed, as those patients will do, I just put on opera and he calmed right down. I am convinced that there is a soothing, healing effect of music. I think that if you had somebody who had never been exposed to much of any kind of music during their lifetime, the effect probably wouldn't be as great. But somebody was always exposed to music and got joy out of it during their earlier life, and then are exposed to it during illness and disease . . . I think it has the effect of stimulating the brain." I would dare to take it a step even further than that—could listening to and learning to play music as a child act as a sort of preventive medicine?

How Music Gets Into the Brain

Music enters the head through an ungainly trumpet-shaped appendage called the ear. Oddly elongated outside and strangely nubbled inside, the ear gathers sound and funnels it to a delicate body part called the eardrum, properly known as the tympanic membrane, which is just a stretched piece of skin designed to vibrate when sound waves hit it. When we cup our hand to our ear to hear something better, we're just artificially making our ear bigger to gather in even more sound. Apart from being told by our parents and doctors never to stick Q-tips into our ear canals because we might rupture our eardrums, we rarely give them a thought.

Sound waves vibrate the eardrum, which conducts sound via three tiny bones—the smallest in the human body. The cochlea houses the Organ of Corti and its thousands of hair cells—this is the structure that that gave Dr. Pauker so much trouble in the last chapter. These hair cells respond to sound vibrations at differing frequencies: they turn music into electrical impulses which are flashed back via the tympanic nerve deep into the brain. There are two tympanic nerves, one for each ear, transmitting sound with the infinitely small difference caused by one ear being slightly apart from the other. So the brain receives music already in stereo.

I'm going to let Dr. Psyche Loui take it from here, since this is her area of expertise. She's going to get a little technical here, but don't let the names inhibit you. She explains clearly what each thing does. "The nerve impulse goes through a seven-point pathway in the auditory brainstem. First it goes to the Dorsal Cochlear Nucleus. Then there's the Medial Superior Olive and the Lateral Superior Olive [named for their shape]. These are very important in localizing sounds. They work together to compare sounds from left and right ear. If the sound is coming from left it should hit the left ear slightly earlier and louder than it hits the right ear. They can map that difference and indicate the direction of the sound.

"After that there is the Lateral Lemniscus, which is important in detecting amplitude modulation—changes in loudness. If there is some ambient sound in the background and that suddenly changes levels, our brain needs to know that. It is important from an evolutionary point of view. It is important for someone to quickly orient to that.

"The Inferior Colliculus is important for harmony. Two tones that interact and sound dissonant together activate the Inferior Colliculus, but two tones that sound consonant do not. For example if I play a minor second like a C and D-flat, they won't sound good together, and that tends to activate the Inferior Colliculus. Two tones that interact and sound dissonant together activate the inferior colliculus but two tones that sound consonant do not, like if I played a major third.

"Then there is the Thalamus and the Medial Geniculate Body which are important for sending signals to the cortex. After the level of the auditory cortex, neural responses to sound are definitely more sensitive to top-down modulations such as how much attention you are paying to the sound or how well you remember that sound, or how emotionally salient those sounds are.

"The Auditory Cortex is in the superior part of the brain's temporal lobe. The brain has the temporal lobe, which is on the sides of head, and the frontal lobe, which is behind the forehead. The Auditory Cortex is a little bit above the ear on both sides."

Right about here, music makes the leap into the soul. The soul being defined as the construct that is the sum of our heritage as primates, plus the sum of all experiences in our life that we recall, either consciously or unconsciously . . . plus something eternal and something connected to a Higher Power, if we want to go there. The Auditory Cortex distributes the musical nerve impulses to the parts of the brain that compare it with past experiences, activate memories, activate associations that make us feel happy or sad or awed—the part of the brain that balances the necessities of eating, sleeping, procreating, and dealing with other people against a sense of mortality and a barely glimpsed awareness of infinity and the eternal.

For each of us, that piece of music might differ—for some, like Michael Barnett, it is Bach; for others it may be the "Ode to Joy" section of Beethoven's Ninth Symphony, or even a childhood lullaby. Dr. Nicholas E. Tawa Jr., a violist and general surgeon at Beth Israel Hospital Medical Center, waxes poetic: "We've all experienced one of those mysterious spiritual and physiological events, a musical moment that crystallizes in an inexplicable beauty in one's brain. It is almost impossible to fathom what the elements are that come together. It's a mystical, nonverbal event that I am convinced has a biological basis."

And it all happens over the distance of about an inch of tissue between the ear and the cortex in that miraculous organ, the brain.

Dr. Loui said she and her colleagues have scanned people's brains while they were listening to music and while they were feeling strong emotions created by the music. "We typically find that areas that are important for action, for initiating motor responses are also active when listening to music, especially music that you know and that you can play. Even if you aren't actually moving your hands, you will form the same brain commands that you would if you were about to initiate those movements.

"Among the regions we find active is the amygdala, which is important for emotional responses. If you take the amygdala out of a bull, the bull won't charge. It is important for forming strong emotional responses such as fear, and it aids in learning that something that is frightening takes priority, which is important for evolutionary reasons. We also see activation of a brain area called the insula, which is important for emotional responses such as disgust and also for encoding voice.

"Those fMRI studies are very important, but we're trying to go even further, to discover not only what parts of the brain are active while listening to music, but how these parts of the brain are communicating with other brain regions, and how they work together to form our complex response to music.

"People talk about the left brain as the analytical side and the right brain as the creative," Dr. Loui said. "That has been shown to be an oversimplification of the complex workings of the brain. It's not that medicine uses the left brain and music uses the right; it's the fact that medicine uses *both* sides of the brain in a unique way, as does music."

In musician/neuroscientist Daniel Levitin's book, *This Is Your Brain on Music*, Levitin concurs with Dr. Loui's observations. He asserts that "the real story is somewhat more nuanced." While certain aspects of music, such as identifying a piece of music, performer, or instrument, are predominantly processed by the left brain, the right brain may be simultaneously analyzing the contour and melody of the music. And here is where neuroplasticity comes in: the brain is always learning and always changing. New connections are being made every time we hear a piece of music or learn a new song. Levitin points out that children's brains are less lateralized than adult brains, and writes that "musical training appears to have the effect of shifting some music processing from the right (imagistic) hemisphere to the left (logical) hemisphere, as musicians learn to talk about—and perhaps think about—music using linguistic terms." [1]

We wonder why there are so many musicians who show an aptitude in science, engineering, and medicine. It's always been fascinating to me to watch my colleagues in rehearsal, interacting with the conductor and with each other as musicians—but also, subtly, using the skills they have developed as doctors as well—such as high-speed, high-level analysis, decision-making, and cooperation.

Could it be that the structure of the brains of musician-physicians like those in the Longwood Symphony Orchestra have been developed from their many years of training as musicians? In 1995, Gottfried Schlaug, Lutz Jäncke, and colleagues showed that the corpus callosum, a collection of neural connections that act as an "information highway" linking the left and right hemispheres, is thicker in musicians, as we saw in Chapter Seven. Their work also suggests that these changes to the Corpus Callosum are a *result* of musical training.[2]

MUSIC ON THE BRAIN

The intersection between science, music, and patient care has attracted the curiosity of some of the brightest minds in the LSO. Colleagues Andrea Spencer, Michael Barnett, and Psyche Loui organized two biannual symposia on the subject, bringing together researchers, philosophers, teachers, therapists, and other educators to exchange ideas, appropriately entitled "Crossing the Corpus Callosum: Neuroscience, Healing and the Arts." These are people who are involved in using innovative art and music curricula to teach people about things we wouldn't normally associate with the arts. Drs. Joel Katz and Shah Khoshbin teach Harvard Medical students "visual literacy"and the art of physical diagnoses by teaching them art observation exercises at the Museum of Fine Arts.[3] Scientists like Dr. Laurel Trainor and Nadine Gaad are studying the effect of music on people with traumatic brain injury and children with autism. We also include children in normal development for education. Among the leaders in the field is neurologist and organist Gottfried Schlaug of Beth Israel Deaconess Medical Center. Then there are Daniel J. Levitin and Robert Zatorre, who are part of a group at McGill University in Montreal examining at this research. It's actually a very big, interesting, and active field. We have so much to learn about the brain and how we process language and emotion.

One of the mysteries is the fact that people seem to use different parts of the brain for talking and for singing. Barnett said, "Though singing seems to be just another kind of language, it apparently uses completely different pathways in the brain. People who have suffered brain injury through trauma or stroke where their language centers are damaged or even missing, often then can still sing. Through music and other arts like theater you are using a different part of your brain. You are using different pathways which enable you to be more creative and more insightful and I would think that research is going to show us that we can gain a lot of intellectual flexibility and power from really engaging the arts more effectively and learning how to use them in patient care, especially in neurology.

"One of the great things that we've learned in the symposia that we've done on music and the brain is that music has a profound influence and involvement in multiple brain areas and circuits. We have discovered that many of those circuits run parallel to other processes we use in our daily life: speaking, acting, et cetera. There's something very powerful about having a way of expressing oneself in a completely parallel way to what we view as our normal mode. In rehab you try to teach people with brain trauma or sickness to speak again. Music gives them another way to express themselves and to regain access to damaged areas which have prevented them from speaking or behaving normally."

We've seen how the brain absorbs and processes music, and we've seen how the musician–physician's brain works. But now let's take a look at some of the ways music interacts with the malfunctioning brain.

9

Overcoming Discord

PERHAPS THE MOST MARVELOUS THING about the brain is how smoothly and quietly it does so many complex things. Its malfunctions are rare, but interesting, especially when they involve the way we process music.

Given the ubiquity of music in human culture, one of the most interesting challenges for music researchers is the phenomenon of tone deafness—the inability to discriminate between different pitches. As this book was being written, Dr. Psyche Loui was in the midst of working on a five-year grant to explore the causes of this affliction.

"Most people can hear pitch differences much smaller than one semitone," she said. "That lets you tune to an orchestra or to a chamber group. But between four and ten percent of people can't hear any difference between, say, an A and a

B-flat, and it's most noticeable when they try to sing. These people are remarkably not good at singing.

"We have some brain imaging studies with good results so far, showing that actually a lot of the brain regions that are deficient in people who are tone deaf are shared with language regions. The classic party line was that the Left Hemisphere is responsible for language and Right Hemisphere is for music. It turns out that it is more complicated than that. There are sort of islands of brain regions that are important in perceiving and producing sounds that are important for pitch and also for speech.

"The Broca's and Wernicke's areas are the classic names for areas that have been shown to be useful in both speech and pitch in music. Technically known as the inferior frontal gyrus, Broca's area is named after the neurologist Paul Broca, who found that if you don't have an inferior frontal gyrus (due to stroke or brain injury, for instance), you can't talk fluently. The other important area that is traditionally known to be important in speech comprehension is the superior temporal gyrus, known as Wernicke's area. We found that Broca's area and Wernicke's area are less well-connected in the tone-deaf individual. In fact, out of ten tone-deaf individuals that we looked at, there seemed to be one branch of this connection called the arcuate fasciculus that we did not detect at all in tone-deaf people that we did detect in controls. It seems that they either have it missing or it was so abnormal that with current imaging techniques we could not detect it.

But is this nature or nurture? Likely both. "I think it has something to do with brain development. If you don't get enough exposure to pitched information early in life, you might not develop those necessary pathways for fine-tuning pitch production and perception.

"We've got another project just starting on Absolute Pitch. Absolute Pitch is the ability to categorize a pitch without a reference tone, for instance if you hear a note in isolation and are very sure that it is an A. Most people can't do that without a reference tone. I have it. It seems to be very common among musicians—people with early musical training in particular— and also among people of certain ethnic groups, hinting that genetics may be involved as well. East Asians are more likely to have it than other groups. People with family members who have it are more likely to have Absolute Pitch."

WHISTLING IN THE DARK

You probably know actor and singer Mandy Patinkin as the revenge-bent Inigo Montoya in the film *The Princess Bride*, but he is actually an accomplished stage actor and a huge classical music aficionado. He addressed the issue of mind and music in a special edition of the Public Radio International show "Gray Matters." His subject was "Music and the Brain," which sought to discover "how a symphony or song can shape us and move us and even help define us as human beings."[1]

He quoted neuroscientist Jaak Panksepp, professor of psychobiology at Ohio's Bowling Green State University, who researched what kinds of music produce chills down the spine. He said "The chills occur when the music suddenly shifts, and a single voice, . . . like a lonely, anguished cry in the wilderness . . . emerges from the background."

He speculated that this physical sensation is produced by neurochemicals released by the brain under certain, very specific circumstances. "The most primitive sound is the sound of a child that is lost or distressed, a child that cries. This has to have a powerful, powerful emotional response on the nervous system of the caretaker and we think that this primitive process is the one that might be captivated by those moving passages of music that produce chills."

The show examined the unusual case of Broadway conductor and classical cellist Shepard Coleman who suffered a ruptured artery in the brain that left him in a coma for days. Brain surgery to repair the aneurysm saved his life, but all the bleeding had damaged his brain in an usual way. As he began his recovery, he found that his emotional responses to music had been enormously amplified.

"I hear more," Coleman said on the program. "My awareness is heightened. The intensity of my reaction is heightened."

Coleman identified a duet in Puccini's opera *Madame Butterfly* between Cio-Cio San and her handmaiden. The beauty of that passage had become so intense, it was actually painful for him to hear.

Despite the physical pain and the massively heightened sensitivity to music, Coleman told Patinkin that his extraordinary "handicap" has vastly enriched his life. "I wouldn't have it any other way. I wish I could do it again. I'd love to increase it again by the same increment. . . . If the question is would I rather go back to the way it was before, the answer is an unqualified no."

WILLIAMS SYNDROME

While Coleman's hypersensitivity to music was acquired after a stroke, there are some congenital syndromes that also feature a hightened awareness to music. Dr. Susan Pauker, the violinist geneticist, sees a similar phenomenon in the children she cares for, who have Williams Syndrome (also known as the Williams–Beuren syndrome), a rare genetic defect that causes characteristic physical features such as a curved fifth finger, an elfin face, cognitive deficits, a hyperfocus on others' eyes in social situations, and narrowing of the great vessels of the heart, and is caused by genetic deletion on chromosome 7.[2] Many people with Williams Syndrome are also extraordinarily sociable—and extraordinarily musical.

The Williams Syndrome Association quoted Glenn Schellenberg, Professor of Psychology at the University of Toronto, as saying "The prevalence of Absolute Pitch among people with Williams Syndrome may also be higher than it is among typically developing individuals." In many cases they are unable to read or write text, yet are able to play and sing at a professional level. One Williams patient on the West Coast was able to conduct an orchestra despite barely being able to read. Lyric soprano Gloria Lenhoff, who has been described as a "musical savant," has performed with classical orchestras, not just singing, but accompanying herself on the accordion.

Children with Williams Syndrome respond especially well to music therapy and are able to master a variety of academic skills, which are enhanced if linked in some way with music during the learning process.

MUSICOPHILIA

One of the best recent books on the subject of music and the brain is Dr. Oliver Sacks' masterful 2007 best-seller *Musicophilia: Tales of Music and the Brain*, a collection of anecdotes from his own files and a survey of case studies from around the world about unusual ways music interacts with the mind. A musician–physician himself, Sacks is a professor of neurology and psychology at Columbia University Medical Center, a pianist, and the author of nearly a dozen books, including his classics *The Man Who Mistook His Wife for a Hat* and *Awakenings*, the latter of which was filmed with Robin Williams.

Sacks' *Musicophilia* opens with the story of a surgeon, Dr. Tony Cicoria, who survives being struck by lightning and soon discovers an enhanced, almost obsessive desire to listen to, compose, and play piano music, even though he had never played before. In addition, he found himself "hearing" pieces of music playing ceaselessly inside his head. The effect, termed "hypermusia" or "musicophilia," is described as "a drastic transformation from being vaguely interested in music to being passionately excited by music and in continual need of it."

Among many other stories of "musical misalignments," Sacks chronicles a patient with severe form of amnesia that renders him unable to remember anything for more than a few seconds—except music. And he examines people who suffer from "amusia," an affliction that goes beyond tone-deafness to a place where they cannot recognize or comprehend musical tones at all.

One of Dr. Sacks' colleagues in New York, a leading figure in the field of music therapy, is Dr. Concetta M. Tomaino, co-founder and executive director of the Institute for Music and Neurologic Function. She specializes in using music to treat illnesses of the brain, especially degenerative neurological diseases like Parkinson's and Alzheimer's, and brain damage from accidents and other trauma.

Dr. Tomaino's work is well respected in the scientific world. Equally importantly, she, like Dr. Sacks, has started to make neuroscience understandable to the lay public. In a recent interview on Caring.com, a public health website, Dr. Tomaino explains how music can help neurologic recovery. "If you're trying to get someone with a traumatic brain injury or a stroke or Alzheimer's to walk, and you tell them, 'Lift your legs and walk like this,' it's a difficult concept for them. And if they have to plan how the left foot is moving in relation to the right foot, they have to think about where their body is in space and how to lift up their leg and put it down, and take steps. However, when they're doing this to music, the rhythm provides the structure within which they move. And because they're following the music, they're not thinking about lifting each leg individually. It's almost as if they're using past memories of how to move with music."[3]

ESCAPING THE JAIL OF SILENCE

Unlike the visual cortex or the auditory cortex, there is no single music center in the brain. We know that when you listen to music or play music, you recruit many different parts of the brain to process the whole experience. Which is why it's very interesting that some people who have suffered strokes and can no longer talk can still sing. They are taught to speak again through recruiting the undamaged parts of their brain that they use to sing in order to help them speak again. This is called Music Intonation Therapy, or MIT. One recent success story of MIT's use was in the recovery of Congresswoman Gabrielle Giffords. Following a traumatic brain injury from a gunshot, Giffords lost her ability to speak, but could still sing. She credits Music Intonation Therapy in helping her regain her speech.

But what about speech that is not absent, but disordered? Taro Alexander, the founder and executive director of Our Time, the New York-based theatre troupe for people who stutter, said "Despite what your Aunt Mary and TV 'experts' say, there is really no 'cure' for stuttering. It's a brain-wiring issue, and different stutterers have different brain-wiring issues. So, you see, there is not likely ever to be a single magic bullet that cures stuttering. But the brain has many wires and many kinds of wires. Researchers have found that the parts of the brain that process music and singing are actually different from the ones used in speech.

"At Our Time we make the most of that. We don't try to cure the kids' stutter. We help them escape from the jail of silence that most of the world wants to put them in. We do that in several ways. Most importantly, we give kids the time and patience to get up on stage and say whatever they want to say in whatever time it takes to say it, without anyone telling them to 'hurry up' or 'slow down' or 'just relax' or by finishing their sentences for them. Many of the kids also sing a lot and write their own songs. Singing is a wonderful way to express oneself. The other fun thing about singing is that most people who stutter don't stutter when they sing. Acting, singing, per-forming, participating in post-show talk-back sessions with the audience, all of these activities help build their confidence and show the world that they can communicate and communicate powerfully and clearly, even if they stutter."

Even when the brain malfunctions, music sometimes has a miraculous ability to help. Given that music affects so many areas of the brain at once, one can think of a myriad of potential applications, from restoring speech and movement to improving reading and communication. We have only begun to scratch the surface.

$\boxed{10}$

Musician, Heal Thyself

DR. BILL KATES, WHO PLAYS oboe, English horn, and oboe d'amore in the LSO, is a large avuncular man with a full-face beard, wire-framed glasses, and the warm, burly voice and easy smile that make you want to tell him everything. His openness and gentleness are perfect for his profession as a psychiatrist. He has a good sense of humor and a deep-seated affection for humanity.

Bill is a self-described old-timer, having joined the LSO with me after saying good-bye to his friend Maestro Endel Kalam. In fact, it was Bill who administered CPR on stage that fateful night at the Longy School when Kalam died on the podium.

Bill always loved music as a child. But a traumatic event when he was six or seven put him on the double track toward medicine as well. "I was always very frightened about dying," he said. "And then one day two huge dogs chewed up a couple of kids who lived on my block. So my seven-year-old brain formed a plan. I decided I was going to become a doctor and I was going to find—ready for this?—a *cure for death*. That was how I started out in medicine. It turned out to be a little harder than I expected. So, I later modified my ambition and resolved to become a brain surgeon because that was the most difficult thing you could be, and you could actually save lives, which is as close to curing death as you can realistically get."

Kates never had a similar dream about being a musician, but there was music all around him, and he went with the flow. He took piano lessons until age eleven. Then, when his family moved from Michigan to Oklahoma, he took up the oboe, "because my father wanted me to socialize and meet girls and the local band needed an oboist." There in Oklahoma, he met the first of several inspiring oboe teachers that have shaped his life as a musician, continuing on into the present.

From then on, the musical urge put up a good fight with medicine for his attention. When Kates was accepted to Harvard Medical School, his parents gave him four hundred dollars they had saved up so he could buy a good microscope. Torn, Kates finally decided instead to use the four hundred dollars to buy a better oboe. "So I began medical school with a nice oboe and the world's crappiest monocular rented microscope."

He eventually abandoned his ambition to become a brain surgeon and became more interested in how the brain worked. Now he saves lives in a more holistic way, as a psychiatrist.

"Being a musician has helped me as a psychiatrist, no question," said Dr. Kates. "There are a lot of times in my psychiatric office when I find that words are not sufficient. Words can, in fact, be limiting. Words lose their power in those moments of intense feeling you often have with patients. So when those moments come, I wonder how I can express feeling without physical contact. Music! I sometimes sing with my patients. The spiritual 'Sometimes I Feel Like a Motherless Child' is wonderful to sing to someone in your office if they are feeling just that.

"It depends on the circumstances. I've even sung Gilbert & Sullivan songs: 'And everyone will say/ As he walks his mystic way/ Oh what a very very very fine young man/ This fine young man must be.' I sometimes sing that to someone when they're talking about how much they want to be loved and how special they need to be.

"Music helps me, too," he continued. "When I'm disturbed, when I'm upset, when I feel inadequate in my work, when I feel cut off from my feelings, music takes me to an almost guaranteed place of openness and nurturance. After I fractured my elbow and worried if I would ever play the oboe again, I used Bach to repair, Schütz to pray with, and Schubert to cry with. That was the sequence. Friday mornings, at the end of my week, that's when I play Bach obbligatos. Even if I have something else to prepare for the LSO, I set aside time to play the obbligatos. They make me feel renewed and taken care of, and in contact with something beyond myself— something beyond my limited world. This music, like the music of Jewish prayer, is a place where I feel I can have some contact with the divine."

In way, for Bill, music is a kind of cure for death after all.

Training the Senses

"There's nothing that trains your senses better than the arts. Nothing," said Dr. Sheldon, the radiation oncologist who sits next to Dr. Kates in the oboe section. "Medicine involves a lot of senses. You have to be able to feel things. You palpate for cancers. You feel the temperature and texture of the skin in general physical examinations. You look into the throat and ears for signs of infection or damage. You have to be able to listen to someone's lungs or heartbeat and hear when something sounds amiss. When people talk to you and describe their symptoms, you have to hear what they are saying to you. I think that the arts are really good for all of that. There's lots of different ways that we learn to connect to our own senses and to other people. I think the more ways we do that, the better."

Shaping the Musician's Brain

A powerful article appeared in the March 2009 issue of *The Journal of Neuroscience* that may shed still more light on the special connection between music and medicine, titled "Musical Training Shapes Structural Brain Development." [1] In a study carried out by an international collaboration of leaders in the field of music and neuroscience, led by Dr. Gottfried Schlaug (a Boston-based organist and a leading expert on the neuroscience of music) and including Drs. Krista Hyde and Ellen Winner, the article asked the question whether neurologic changes and structural brain changes in children who learned a musical instrument were innate or not—the question of "nature" vs. "nurture." In other words, were they born with a proclivity toward music, or was it instilled in them by others? Is there something structurally unique in the brains of children who play music? Or does the playing of music, encouraged by parents, teachers, et al., actually shape children's brains and rewire the way their brains work to make them musical?

The researchers observed that "there is a widespread view that learning to play a musical instrument in childhood stimulates cognitive development and leads to the enhancement of skills in a variety of extramusical areas," and they set out to see if learning to play a musical instrument changed the actual structure of the brain. Two groups of children were matched for age, gender, and socioeconomic status. Over a fifteen-month period, two groups of children (average age six years old) received either weekly half-hour keyboard lessons or forty minutes of group singing and drumming classes, and were studied with neuropsychologic testing and functional MRI.

"The results were compelling and very exciting. We demonstrated regional structural brain plasticity in the developing brain that occurred with only fifteen months of instrumental musical training in early childhood. Structural brain changes in motor and auditory areas (of critical importance for instrumental music training) were correlated with behavioral improvements on motor and auditory–musical tests. This study is the first longitudinal investigation to directly correlate brain structure and behavioral changes over time in the developing brain."

Further, they found that "children who played and practiced a musical instrument showed greater improvements in motor ability (as measured by finger dexterity in both left and right hands) and in auditory melodic and rhythmic discrimination skills."

THESE FINDINGS, ADDED TO THOSE mentioned in previous chapters, point the way to what I have always believed is a special relationship between doctors and their music seen much further down the developmental spectrum.

"I think there are a lot of correlating factors," Dr. Loui the brain researcher said. "You have to have patience to sit through many hours of practice and rehearsal, and to sit through many areas of studying in medical school. Music trains your attention in a way that leads to better practice, better perception, better attention, better memory, which are all important in medical practice. Families who put a lot of money in their children might put them through violin and piano lessons and also might be the families that put them through medical school. I'm not completely comfortable in saying that there is a one-directional causal relation. I don't want to say that it's always definitely musical training that directly leads to being a great doctor, because there are a lot of great musicians that don't end up being doctors. But I think there are a lot of correlating factors. People who end up being accomplished musicians also might possess a lot of the same cognitive perceptual neural characteristics. Enhanced perceptual abilities are important in both. Enhanced prefrontal cognitive characteristics, like attention and memory, are important in both.

"The brain that finds the same delight in a slight aural variation in music might be the same brain that perceives a slight variation in a medical lab finding or a minuscule but significant change in an x-ray. Both disciplines require enormous attention to detail."

SOMETHING YOU CAN'T IGNORE

Every one of us has certain favorite pieces that help us, not only in our personal lives, but in our work as doctors too. I asked some of our LSO doctors to share their favorites and to tell me about the physical, psychological, emotional, and spiritual shifts that occur when practicing both medicine and music.

"It is hard to pick favorites, because I love a lot of music," said Barnett. "I really love Bach. The 'Chaconne' from his Partita No. 2 for unaccompanied violin. It is very beautiful. One of my cardiology professors was giving a presentation and he thought it would be classy if he put some Baroque radio on in the background. And while he was giving his presentation, the 'Chaconne' came on. One of the things I really hate is when some really transcendently beautiful music comes on in the background at a store or somewhere. It's really hard for me to ignore, but I have to ignore it because to really enjoy and absorb it I'd have to enter a meditative space and, of course, you can't do that in a store. So there I was, listening to the 'Chaconne' at this medical presentation. The violinist was coming to one of the biggest climaxes in the movement, arpeggiating up and down, and one of the interns quipped, 'With music like this, it's way easier to work.' He had been trying to tune out the performance up to that point, but the power of a real performance of great music is something you can't ignore."

Barnett has an intense curiosity and interest in how music, music administration and community service all work together. He is equally intrigued by the demographics of health care delivery—almost in parallel to how an orchestra functions in society, he studies how doctors function in the larger medical and social community.

He joined the LSO as a first-year medical student, already with a master's degree in oboe performance from his alma mater, Yale University. As chair of the Community Engagement Committee for the past three years, Michael led his committee in organizing LSO's educational program and formalized the application program for the Healing Art of Music. He will enter his internship in Medicine at Brigham and Women's Hospital in 2011, with an ambition to go into primary care (which is rare in the Harvard world of academia). My guess is he will emerge one of the next generation's leaders in redefining and strengthening the role of the primary care physician—the type of doctor most people come in contact with most often, and thus the type who has the biggest impact on their overall health.

He continues with his list of favorite works with a faraway look as though scanning through his CD collection. "What kind of music touches me?" It seems there are different composers for different moods.

"I love Bach's *Ich Habe Genug* (that's Cantata Number 82) and *St. Matthew's Passion*, and the Mass in B Minor. Pieces I associate particularly with calm and relaxation are the Haydn Cello Concerti in C and D. When I am feeling more moody and I want to vent my anger and annoyance or distraction through some music, I might listen to some more angry

Shostakovich like his Cello Concerto or the eighth String Quartet. The Bartok String Quartets are also very angular and moving. But Schoenberg's *Five Pieces for Orchestra* is also incredibly moving—very deep and brooding. The Brahms symphonies have always been a huge release for me. The third movement of the Third Symphony is one of the most beautiful outpourings of simple romantic beauty in my heart. If I feel the need to be enveloped in a lush blanket of warmth, I might listen to the Fourth Symphony."

A GREAT EQUALIZER

Playing music in an orchestra gives high-intensity doctors a chance to let down their hair around each other a bit and escape for a time from the hierarchical world of the operating room and the academic world. There are no attending physicians, senior residents, or interns—in the orchestra there are only musicians.

Barnett plays first oboe in a woodwind section that includes experienced physicians who are decades his senior. "Tom Sheldon, who is a radiation oncologist, sits to my left playing second oboe, and Daniela Krause sits to my right. She's a leukemia specialist who does transfusion medicine. So I'll be studying for my board exams or my shelf exams and I'll ask him some question that I am trying to figure out. I'll call out, 'Hey Tom. What does L-5 innervate?' Or I'll be going through my little note cards with different beta blocker medications and I'll say, 'Hey Tom, can you remind me of the difference between these two drugs?' or I'll ask Dany some of my questions about diagnosing different blood smears and I'll be looking at slides and she'll point something out and she'll say, 'Oh these are Pelger-Huet cells.' And that's always been really fun.

"We all come from the same world, and that's a huge pleasure for me. Dany and I will be playing through a duet and work out how to do the crescendos or tune together. Or Tom and I will work through something in the same way. We are constantly engaged in the music, but every now and then our medicine sides poke through."

The doctors of the LSO are not above asking for on-the-spot diagnoses either. There was one evening when one of our bass players was having abdominal pain, which turned out to be a gallstone. During break the musicians were heard to be saying "Don't consult the violinist—he's a dermatologist. Not the horn player either, she's an anesthesiologist. Talk to the bassoonist. He's a gastroenterologist—*he'll* know what to do."

"One of the nice things about Longwood Symphony is that the music is a great equalizer," continued Barnett. "We are all in the orchestra together and, in the end, no one is really more or less important as a musician in the orchestra than anyone else. Some people have more prominent roles, but everyone needs to work together to create a beautiful sound."

The same is true in a large hospital. There may be more "glamour" spots, but everyone—from orthopedic surgeons to anesthesiologists to social workers, nurses, and aides—works together to heal the people who come in.

A Symphony of Healing

And Barnett has a theory. Doctors in a modern world filled with specialists need to collaborate like musicians in an orchestra.

"You go to your G.P. with an ailment and she may send you to one doctor for tests, a specialist for one aspect of your ailment, and yet another specialist for another aspect of your ailment. For you to get better, all these doctors must work together. I find they work best when there is a 'chamber music' aspect to the relationship—a small group of specialized talents working tightly and closely together in a way that everyone can hear everyone else and respond instantaneously.

"There's a lot of concern in the health policy world that care is hopelessly fragmented in this country. In my research I have found that's especially true of doctors who take care of Medicare patients. In Boston the average doctor has about a hundred Medicare patients—not an unreasonable figure today, which is perhaps equally shocking. If each of those patients needs care from five specialists over the course of a year, that means that each doctor is potentially coordinating treatment with five hundred other doctors each year, which is pretty staggering.

"But then you have to realize that number is half or even a third as many as other places in the country. Some enlightened places like the Mayo Clinic or Intermountain Health Care in Utah use a chamber music approach. If you have a patient with cancer, there's an ongoing dialogue between the primary care doctor, the oncologist, the radiation oncologist, the surgeon, and then anyone else that needs to be in touch, including the dermatologist who is managing some skin side effect of chemotherapy. They make sure their plans are harmonious—that they're actually working together toward a common goal, rather than everyone tackling their own individual slice of patient care.

"If you have a string quartet or a wind quartet where everyone is just playing their part and not responding to the other, it sounds terrible. Maybe something will come out that resembles a piece of music. But it doesn't *feel* like music. Someone's going to get way more care than they need or something's going to be ignored or there are going to be conflicts, just like in a piece of music where people step on one another's solos, or they are not going to play the same notes the same length, or they are not going to end at the same time. If I'm not being aware of what the conductor is doing or the intonation and dynamics of everyone around me, I'm not going to be a part of the group. I think creating a harmonious health outcome for the patient requires the same coordination.

"And that is something in the Longwood Symphony that we are always working to do better. So that's how my research ties into that narrative. The research itself is another creative, improvisatory endeavor. In scientific research I think it is sometimes not appreciated how creative it is. In fact, sometimes I feel it is only creativity and interpretation. Because when you read a scientific paper, it looks like things are so dry and prescribed. But actually every single sentence implies dozens of decisions that were made and lots of discussion in how to interpret and use prior results and just our feeling of intuition and our understanding of the deep underpinnings of what we are studying to try to move things forward in a logical way that is also a very creative, collaborative endeavor.

"It is the reason why you see, especially in our orchestra, a lot of people who are involved in music, medicine, and research: because they all use slightly different combinations of the same skills of flexibility, creativity, improvisation based on a body of knowledge and experience."

Humanism in Medicine

There is a growing interest nationwide for the next generation of doctors to embrace the humanities. Sandra Gold is executive director of the Arnold P. Gold Foundation, founded by her husband, a neurologist and musician, which promotes humanism in medicine. She is concerned that medicine is becoming more and more the handmaiden of technology. The hands-on healing aspect of medicine is being lost, and a time may come when the younger generation loses contact with that enormously fulfilling aspect of our calling. Many medical students seem to be choosing their specialties based on lifestyle rather than a choice that cares for the most patients or relieves the most suffering or is something that they are intellectually passionate about. Naturally, this has always been a lure for young doctors, but the lure is getting stronger year by year.

To combat that, Humanism in Medicine is teaching young doctors and medical students to give more of themselves, frequently through the arts. The whole mission of that organization is to bring the medical student back to the reason why doctors are doctors.

Medical expression through the humanities may have a part to play in righting this imbalance. Healing—through poetry, drama, and, of course, music—is becoming increasingly accepted as a form of therapy for not only the patients but the healers themselves. With long hours, debt, insurance costs, and the myriad other issues that can plague any working person trying to balance career, family, and the demands of modern life, doctors are often in need of a little healing themselves.

Besides, as Pulitzer Prize-winning composer John Adams said in his commencement speech to the graduating class of The Juilliard School in 2010, "A life in the arts means loving complexity and ambiguity, of enjoying the fact that there are no single, absolute solutions. And it means that you value communicating about matters of the spirit over the baser forms of human interaction, because you know that life is not just a transaction, not simply a game about winning someone's confidence purely for purposes of material gain."

"DANY, YOU'RE BEAMING"

Dr. Daniela Krause, the clinical pathologist whose specialty is blood issues, namely transfusion medicine and leukemia research, also plays flute and piccolo in the Longwood Symphony Orchestra. Born in Berlin, she is tall and slim with blue eyes and curly blonde hair. She speaks with a soft blend of English and German accents, reflecting her dual heritage.

Doctors learn to compartmentalize their feelings. Music, for the musician-physician, provides a healthy arena to let bottled-up feelings flow.

"I'll give you an example," said Dr. Krause. "Imagine for a moment that you are a transfusion-medicine person. You get called at three Sunday morning because somebody has had a terrible car accident and has already used up one hundred units of red cells, about ten doses of platelets, and fifty doses of fresh frozen plasma. You can just imagine what this patient is going to look like. You go in and sometimes their bellies are still open. Well, you can't stand there and cry or wonder how terrible the world is. You have to treat that person. And waiting next is a gunshot victim who has bullets all through him. You will yourself not to cry. But where does all that grief go? You put it into your music. When you play an instrument you feel better."

One of Krause's favorite moments in the LSO came in summer 2010 when we played on the Esplanade beside Boston's Charles River where some nine thousand music lovers gathered on blankets and chairs. When Maestro McPhee threw in a Glenn Miller piece, people got up and danced.

Afterward, Krause recalls, "I walked out of the stage door and a friend of mine from the German consulate said to me 'Dany, you're beaming!' This is what usually happens to me when I play music. I get this big smile on my face. I felt good because I knew we had played really well and because we made nine thousand people happy. When you are a physician you can perhaps make one person happy at a time. But this was nine thousand 'patients' at once. I think reaching out to people en masse like that is pretty amazing. Playing music is like taking care of a patient—except that you can reach so many more people in one go. I think that's especially true for those in the cancer field, where your patients often don't get better. In the long run, though, you are still trying to do something good for them. I think music has exactly the same effect."

TOTALLY HUMAN

For Dr. Buchmiller, that effect comes specifically from Beethoven. "I love Beethoven's Seventh Symphony. It was one of the first big classical pieces I played back when I was thirteen in Youth Symphony, and I still think it tells a beautiful, beautiful story. I also love Beethoven's Ninth, of course. I'm kind of a nut runner; I have it on my iPod and I run to it. The fourth movement is a perfect 5K finish at the end of a long run. If I complete that interval before the final chord, I'm sub 8 and pretty happy. I know every note by heart. Joking aside, the more I play that piece and the more I hear it, the more it brings tears to my eyes. It makes me feel . . . I can only describe it as 'totally human.'"

Music provides a safety valve for doctors, especially those constantly thrust into emotional situations. "I definitely cry about events at work," Dr. Buchmiller said. "I give people hugs. You allow yourself some expression—but you still have to step back a little bit. You can't be ultra-emotional, ultra-invested all the time, otherwise you could risk being ineffective."

For Buchmiller, Beethoven and the world of music help supply that missing emotional piece.

"As a doctor, especially as a doctor of pediatric surgery, I'm confronted with the circle of life every day. In a single week I deal with life, death, birth, celebration, sadness, and so many other emotions. Beethoven's Ninth is a celebration of the entire circle of life. Somehow, Beethoven helps it all fit into the universe a little bit better for me. My parents are getting older and I think, 'My goodness, Dad's eighty-five and Mom's seventy-nine . . . they've had such a great life. They are so healthy.' At the same time I see children in my care at work with such serious challenges. Their lives are in my hands. Sometimes there are miracles, and they are amazing.

But the music allows me to put that somewhere and have peace about it. It lets my brain take a deep breath and find that little space of calm."

TRANSFORMING YOURSELF

Peter Stein is a professional violist turned chiropractor in private practice. He is a tall man with black hair and beard, heavy eyebrows, and blue eyes who peaks with a quiet but resonant baritone voice.

Now a student at Boston University, Stein continues to seek new knowledge in ways to heal: he has recently returned to school to pursue a doctorate degree in Rehabilitation Science, with a focus on human movement.

"Four hundred years ago French philosopher René Descartes said that the mind and the body were two separate things," Stein said, "and many people have been taught to believe that. But so much philosophy and science has come out recently about how the brain and the body interact, that it's bordering on the foolish to keep believing in such a dichotomy."

Each instrument carries with it a certain distinctive set of aches and pains. "I'm not saying everybody using that instrument will feel these symptoms—or will feel any at all," said Dr. Stein. "But by the time the players get to me they tend to present in a certain way. Horn players have jaw problems. String players put a lot of wear and tear on the tendons in their fingers and wrists. Percussionists often have wrist problems from using their mallets on different surfaces and sometimes have back problems as well. Flute players have to bear the weight of the instrument on their hands in addition to fingering the keys. They frequently present with ulnar neuropathy, which is a nerve problem of the fourth and fifth fingers and can lead to numbness and wasting of the hand muscles. A lot of neck problems as well, fairly chronically, because of their posture.

"Bass players can rest their instrument on the floor, but it is one of the largest instruments and the musicians are expected to carry them from gig to gig. At least pianists don't have to worry about moving their instruments! So the bassists have shoulder problems from carrying the instrument and wrist and finger problems from playing. But they have fewer complaints of low back pain than cellists do, because cellists are pinned behind their instruments and have to literally reach over the bulk of the instrument to play."

One of the most frightening ailments a musician faces is called focal dystonia, a neurological problem that causes loss of fine motor coordination when playing. It is neither specific to musical instrument nor musical genre. Some well-known classical musicians with focal dystonia include pianists Leon Fleisher and Gary Graffman, oboist Alex Klein of the Chicago Symphony, and guitarist David Leitner, but there are jazz, bluegrass, and punk rock guitarists, banjo players, and horn players who are similarly afflicted. String players find themselves unable to play short quick notes in certain patterns. Horn players lose the ability to make tiny, necessary adjustments of their embouchure. And pianists find that their fingers curl unnaturally into their palm just as they are trying to reach to play a chord.

Many musicians with focal dystonia have been forced to give up or significantly curtail their careers, performing in a limited or altered way. Thankfully, there are many brilliant piano works written for left hand alone. After Austrian concert pianist Paul Wittgenstein (1887-1961) lost his right arm in battle during the First World War, he dedicated himself to commissioning and premiering music by such well-known composers of the twentieth century as Ravel, Hindemith, Britten, Prokofiev, and Korngold. Following Wittgenstein's death in 1961, the music became available to the public. Thanks to his vision, pianists Leon Fleischer and Gary Graffman, both afflicted with focal dystonia of the right hand, have been able to continue performing and championing this unique and diverse body of work.

"Focal dystonia has to do with the way the central nervous system processes movements," explains Dr. Stein. "You get someone doing something very fine and coordinated and complicated enough, and maybe throw a little tendon injury into the mix to force it to become even more complicated and it seems the brain becomes overwhelmed. There are neuroscientists and researchers in other fields such as Physical Therapy professor Nancy Byl who have made the study of focal dystonia their life's work. Using primate studies, they are only just starting to develop models that capture some of what *may* be happening in the process of focal dystonia. There's evidence from her work that some finger control areas of the brain's motor cortex lose their distinctiveness from each other, or become 'smeared.' At some point, the brain stops being able to process all the discrete motor components that go into playing music. Next thing you know the musician tries to lift, say, his fourth finger, and the fifth finger goes along with it. Or maybe he tries to move one knuckle of the fifth finger and the whole thing claws."

Stein continues, contemplatively, "I think it's safe to say that this observation just touches *one* neural level (cortex), whereas it might well be that this disordered process, like motor control itself, is broadly distributed *through* the nervous system, and we have as yet no real concept of most of it . . . that's the really humbling part to contemplate, as I think of it.

"For some of these things, there *is* no cure. You can effect big turnarounds sometimes, but it doesn't feel like effecting a cure. It feels like pulling somebody back from a cliff and saying, 'There's always going to be a cliff there. I want you to be able to live with a margin between you and the cliff. Always keep it on your left.'

"I had a viola player who came to me with a good deal of pain developing in his upper back and his neck. It had gotten to where his neck actually clicked when he moved back and forth. When he played it was easy enough to see why. He would twist himself around the instrument, but I'm not sure he even realized he was doing it. Normally, as we mature, we learn to move in a pretty coordinated way. But when we come upon a specialized object like a musical instrument, we're willing to give some of that up in order to live in the instrument's space. So my job was to find a way for him to use the instrument in a healthy way, to have a physical center, without losing the skill he'd acquired or his emotional relationship with his instrument. You can't take those away from a person, but there are things you can do to make them more comfortable and less destructive.

"I ask my musician patients to bring their instrument and play for me. At some point I will say, 'Freeze! Don't move! I'm a violist, I know what I'm doing. Now . . . I'm going to take your viola away. Don't move while I do it.' The viola comes away and they can feel that they've got their chin stuck out this way, their neck twisted that way. I've seen some funny postures. I almost don't have to say anything before they realize what the point is. They can feel the difference when they don't have the instrument to support. And I say 'If you're not going to be comfortable living like this, we've got to try something different.'

"In the case of the violist, we worked from finding a comfortable balancing point for his neck to finding a way for him to stand so the center of gravity was inside his body and not in his viola. There was a huge turnaround and an enormous reduction in pain. He was one of my more dramatic responses."

Dr. Stein speaks as one who began as an accomplished, professional musician, then retooled his mind to become a respected doctor, and is now retooling it yet again, planning to become a research scientist.

"Every time you learn to do something reasonably well, you have to transform yourself," he said. "Now I'm trying to learn to become a good scientist. That's proving to be hugely transformative for me. Every time you try to do something like that, you find that you become a different person—hopefully a richer, more able person. It also gives you the ability to see the things you already know in a new way. When you turn back to your music, you find things in it you didn't see before. You don't just play the music; while you play, you think about the people who made the music and the people who are listening to it. As a doctor it makes you more compassionate and more understanding. You see people differently the way you see music differently."

He continues, "I can't say I apply music professionally the way a music therapist would. That whole field has slowly been coming into its own, but I admit that I do not have in-depth knowledge about it. I know music therapists say they are seeing transformative results in Parkinson's disease and Alzheimer's. The changes they see when patients listen to music are surprising. There is no question that something is happening there."

But there is one thing Stein is very willing to go out on a limb to state: "For many people—and I fit in here—music is one of the things that make it all worth living through. It's one of the great friends in life."

11

Music and Mental Health

OCCUPATIONAL THERAPIST, TAMARA GOLDSTEIN HAS structured her life around health—her own as well as her patients, and music provides her with the balance she needs so that she can care for others. "Music helps me maintain my health, mentally and physically," Goldstein said. "A large part of my work is mental. But when I sit down to play music, I feel like I'm using a completely different part of my brain. The feeling of relief is indescribable. I sit in my chair, the baton goes up, and I mentally ready myself. I'm aware there are people around me because I need to be. But when I play, it feels very much like I'm in my own little world. It's still just me and the music.

"You don't have to play an instrument to feel there is a rhythm to life. Music is everywhere. We surround ourselves with it every chance we get. Think about that! Whether it's at church, a funeral, a birthday party, exercise, a New Year celebration, or just to unwind when you come home from work. It helps us to be in harmony with the rest of the world. We all try to achieve harmony. When we're out of harmony with life, we can sense it. In Italian they say *stonato,* you're out of tune. Music helps us regain and maintain that natural rhythm in all our lives."

The Ballad of Ruth

"I'm often sent to dementia units, which can be spooky. You see people silently wandering. They don't make eye contact. They appear to be empty shells of their former selves. I once was asked to see a lady named Ruth who had fallen and fractured her hip. She was in a unit located in an old historical building in Boston, an old-fashioned Victorian. The unit was located on the top floor with a low ceiling. Reserved as the 'dementia unit,' it felt like a deliberate separation or distancing from the rest of the population both inside the building and from the community outside. You could practically see the cobwebs. The atmosphere is sobering and instantly provokes a sad and haunting feeling of the loss of one's self."

After all, who are "we" without our memories and experiences? Ruth seemed to have completely lost her memories, and with them, her "self."

"When I would go to see Ruth she always seemed to be asleep in her chair. Her eyes were always closed. Physical Therapy didn't want to go near her. They said, 'One service is enough. She's gone.' It was my job to take her to the rehab department in her wheelchair every day and try to elicit some kind of response.

"The first day, I tried putting cold water on her face. Nothing. I tried warm water. Nothing. I tried calling her: 'Ruth! Ruth! Hello!' And again she just sat there. Following the requirements of the insurance company, I did that for an hour every day. She was alive, but completely unresponsive. It felt like an exercise in futility.

"So, to make it a little more interesting for myself, I started to talk to her. I'd chatter away, but no response. It was a way to pass the time and it did her no harm.

"Finally one day, I was being super animated and she was just sitting there with her head slumped sideways and her eyes closed, like always. And I said, 'Let's turn on the radio and see what's on WCRB,' Boston's classical station. The music came on and I said, as it was playing, 'Ruth, I'd like to know a little more about you. Do you like classical music? I play the violin in the Longwood Symphony Orchestra. I think that's kind of impressive.'

"And suddenly she raised her head and opened her eyes. It was like a doll being wound up after sitting on a shelf. Everyone in the room got quiet. Ruth looked at me and said 'My husband was a composer.' It was the first time she had spoken in months, if not years.

"Everyone asked me, 'What did you do?' I said, 'I just turned on the radio.'

"They ran into the office and Googled her name and found that her husband really WAS a composer! I said, 'Ruth what about you? Do you like music?'

"As if nothing had happened during those silent months, she looked up and said 'I was an opera major at the New England Conservatory. Would you like to hear me sing?'

"And in this clear soprano she began singing, '*The hills are alive with the sound of music. . . .*'

"That song has so many beautiful, touching lyrics. It turned out that Ruth had a very nice voice indeed. She started walking. She would sing and smile as she walked. She told us she had started a music camp and it's still in operation. We looked it up and found that nothing she was telling us was false or fabricated. I couldn't believe it was the same woman.

"After that, she seemed remarkably able to accept her environment. Music didn't 'cure' her, but the change in her demeanor was as though a switch had been turned on. She was interacting and participating in simple everyday activities again. It felt like a miracle. The music may have been just the right kind of connection she required, perhaps a combination of stimulating interest with something that was meaningful to her from her distant past, the familiar sounds of music emanating from the radio and the stimulation of her brain by soothing sounds may have awakened neuropathways and neurochemicals that aroused her to consciousness. There is no doubt for me that music facilitated her ability to heal."

TERRITORIES IN THE MIND

Looking back at her story about Ruth, many people would consider Goldstein's working world a stressful or even depressing place to be. Some of her patients in the later stages of Alzheimer's suffer from significant neurological conditions. Sometimes the rooms are cramped and airless. But to Goldstein, these are places where she can help people feel better and where many of her patients find a connection with one another, as well as with her, despite the limitations that illness, disease, disability, and age may have placed on them. She is able to help people no one else can (or wants to) help. She looks for the hope and joy in healing.

"My job as an occupational therapist is, for example, to understand what a hip replacement is, and what you need to do, according to scientific studies, to help you recover ability and resume as many of your normal physical activities as possible. But another part of what I do is to find out who you are, what you like, what makes *you* feel better. I look at the whole person. Ultimately my job is to help people feel less burdened by their illness and suffering, even if I can't completely eliminate it, and to help them to return to living with the least amount of restrictions or professional support, for an environment of their choice."

On Thursday evenings, Tamara Goldstein carries her violin into the Boston Latin School, transforming herself from occupational therapist to violinist as she climbs the stairs to the band room. Even if she has been emotionally drained that day, she finds solace in her music. Music helps to heal the healer. "I believe that I was born with a high degree of sensitivity," she said. "For whatever complex set of reasons, music affects me deeply. I am drawn to it. I like that I can create a mood by choosing a genre of music, a style of music, a tempo, a tone, an instrument or orchestration. I like that I can fully submit to music and let it lead me by my emotions wherever it wants to take me. I like that it can provoke a memory. I like that it creates images and scenes in my mind and that it can fire my imagination.

"There are emotional territories in which the music navigates through my mind, my heart, my spirit, and my soul.

Some of those territories have valleys of sadness, and some lift me to peaks of lightness. Music doesn't stay in just one territory; it is nomadic. It can shift from my mind to my heart to my soul and to my spirit. As my arms work the bow and the fingerboard I can feel the music flowing through my complex inner emotional history. Tears rise up from the depths, sometimes from the intensity of the delicate beauty, sometimes from the intensity of the awe it creates, sometimes from the intensity of the sadness, and sometimes from the pain.

"And when I finish the piece, my consciousness of everything else around me will suddenly return."

MUSIC IN HOSPITALS

With improving research and the advocacy by such organizations as the Society for Arts in Healthcare and the American Music Therapy Association, the movement to incorporate music into our prescription for healing is growing. Case studies like Ruth's are finding their way into scholarly journals that document the effects of music on mental health, from dementia to mood disorders.

A 2009 clinical trial in Canterbury, U.K., concluded that anxiety levels in patients scheduled for endoscopy were significantly reduced by listening to music.[1] A group of studies surveyed by *Therapy Times* found that music helped improve symptoms for patients as young as four and as old as ninety-eight on a range of physical and mental health issues from grief to pain to cancer.[2]

As useful as recorded music is during procedures, the power of live music on patients has been observed by doctors for decades. Music in Hospitals, a U.K. organization, has been in existence for more than sixty years. Professional musicians give performances in hospitals, hospices, daycare centers, and other healthcare and special education facilities. In 2009, MiH sent out musicians for more than five thousand such concerts, finding that "Sharing the experience of a live musical performance can help reduce levels of anxiety, pain and depression."[3]

MUSICORPS

In January 2011, the Longwood Symphony Orchestra invited classically trained performer and composer Arthur Bloom to Boston to participate in our "Crossing the Corpus Callosum" symposium on music, neuroscience, and healing. Bloom works with severely injured Iraq War veterans at Walter Reed Army Medical Center in a program he created called Musicorps. Professional musicians work with young men and women recovering from severe war injuries, challenging them with intense musical training to confront their pain and anger through performance and song-writing. In most cases, these soldiers are not playing traditional classical instruments, but electric guitars and keyboards. Some of these patients are double and triple amputees; most are suffering from post-traumatic stress disorder. Bloom works with physical therapists and prosthetics engineers to create artificial limbs that accommodate their disabilities. Bloom recounts that many of these individuals have impatiently rejected further physical and occupational therapy, yet will willingly practice several hours a day. Through music, the program urges the soldiers to engage with their pain and often with their anger, to explore and release emotions helping them to cope with their PTSD symptoms as well.

There are many programs around the country like Musi-corps that engage injured veterans in intensive music programs, sometimes adapting musical instruments to accommodate their injuries. Arthur has related that, when regarded as musicians, the veterans will spend hours practicing intricate fingerwork, strumming technique, or rhythm practice. These are the same war-weary vets who will sometimes resist traditional physical and occupational therapy.

The high-level training and hours of practice stimulate neurological recovery in soldiers who have suffered injuries to the brain, improving their memory, ability to concentrate, and executive function. The program also improves their sense of identity and self-esteem, which have usually taken a huge hit. They used to be physically strong, competent, confident soldiers; now they are stuck in a hospital. But in this setting, they are no longer patients but fellow musicians.

Slate columnist Anne Applebaum quoted one of Bloom's Musicorps protegés who referred to the program as "the healing power of Death Metal." Bloom is currently working with Dr. Allen Brown, Director of Brain Research and Reha-bilitation at the Mayo Clinic. Together, they are hoping to replicate the program in other veteran's hospitals across the country. In the meantime, Musicorps has a waiting list of wounded soldiers clamoring to join.[4]

"One of the great things that we learned at the symposium is that music has a profound influence and involvement in multiple brain areas and circuits," said Dr. Michael Barnett. "We have dis-covered that many of those circuits run parallel to other processes we use in our daily life: speaking, acting, et cetera. There's some-thing very powerful about having a way of expressing oneself in a completely parallel way to what we view as our normal mode. In rehab you try to teach people with brain trauma or sickness to speak again. Music gives them another way to express themselves and to regain access to damaged areas which have prevented them from speaking or behaving normally."

MUSICAL HEALTH

Just as the men and women at Musicorps are no longer simply soldiers, veterans, or patients, but musical colleagues with shared experiences, so too the physicians who are musicians cannot be identified as one or the other. Our shared experiences are too tightly intertwined.

So, should people choosing a doctor ask, "Where did you go to school?" "How long have you been practicing medicine?" *and* "What instrument do you play?" They should! Given the high percentage of physicians who are also musicians, they will find that the field hasn't been reduced much, and it might open a more intimate dialogue with your physician along the way, something rarer and rarer in today's health care climate.

What do patients get from it? Something I call "Musical Health"—the tangential healing benefits patients experience when being cared for by musician-physicians.

Dr. Stephen Wright, the bassoonist, has personally experienced the power of music when the tables were turned and he became the patient, in need of a painful arthrogram on an injured shoulder. "The hospital said I should bring a disc of music to listen to," he said. "I brought a recording of a newly discovered bassoon piece and all I remember is the music. It completely distracted me. It was very soothing. I didn't feel anything. I'd say it took thirty or forty minutes, and they were done before the disc was over. It was a very powerful way of shifting my focus away from whatever it is they were doing over there."

Dr. Wright applies that lesson to his own patients. "I use music during colonoscopies with my own patients just the way I myself used music for the arthrogram. The patients are usually sedated for the procedure, but we let them choose the music. I sometimes play Longwood Symphony discs, though when I hear my part coming up that can sometimes be distracting! That reminds me of a story: There was one weekend when the endoscopy suite was broken into. They stole a couple of CD players and *all* of the Longwood Symphony discs! I consider that to be one of the greatest compliments Longwood ever got."

A few years ago, we compiled a CD of excerpts from some of our concerts, titled "The Sounds of Healing," which we distributed to patients and colleagues. When we learned that Senator Edward Kennedy, that great champion of the arts and health care, had been diagnosed with a brain tumor, we sent him a copy of the CD. Later, a staff member close to the senator shared with us that he listened to it often during his many trips between Cape Cod and Massachusetts General Hospital. I can only hope, and believe, that it helped him during his battle with cancer for all those years.

Must it be Music *or* Medicine?

For Dr. Andrea Spencer, still a training resident in psychiatry, the roles of clinician and musician sometime seems to be in direct conflict.

"We go into psychiatry because we love people and find people interesting," she said. "We love treating the whole person. Yet in psychiatry you are not supposed to bring yourself into the patient–doctor relationship, at least not in the same way you would as a primary care physician or even a dermatologist. In other fields of medicine you touch your patients all the time. But in psychiatry, there is a lot of debate whether it is okay to embrace or even touch patients. I hate that rule. It's my instinct to lay a hand on someone's back when it's called for."

It's the same way with music, unfortunately. If you play music for a patient, you're showing them that you know how to play music, which means you are revealing what you do with your free time. That's a no-no for psychiatrists—for good reason in many cases, but still limiting. However, when I treat them in my own practice as a pediatrician, I do ask my patients what kind of music they listen to, and that is not just out of curiosity. I find that that kind of knowledge can help a doctor both diagnostically and therapeutically. Imagine meeting someone who says they do not listen to *any* music *ever*, versus somebody who has a strong opinion about music. Those are two very different people. It will tell you a lot about their ability to feel, their motivations, and about their ability to engage with the world. This is something Dr. Spencer can make use of, too.

"For some people, avoiding music is a protective mechanism," she said. "Music can make you feel strong emotions, and some people don't want to feel those emotions. You can't tell people to listen to sad music to purge their sadness because some people won't be able to handle it. But there are other patients for whom sad music can provide an amazing catharsis. If you want to use music as a therapy, you have to tailor it carefully to the patient. It could actually be helpful in their therapy."

HEALING THE HEALERS—LSO ON CALL

A few years ago, the Longwood Symphony began a monthly chamber music outreach program, "LSO on Call." It gives musicians from the orchestra the opportunity to perform as small ensembles in hospitals and other patient care facilities, bringing music to those who, for a variety of reasons, cannot attend our regular concerts in Jordan Hall. These moving experiences have frequently proved as therapeutic to the medical musicians themselves as to the patients and their families.

Dr. Andrea Spencer was one of the creators of LSO on Call. As a psychiatrist in training, she is particularly attuned to the impact these performances have on all involved, and was particularly moved by her own experience in the program.

Last year, at the end of a grueling three-month rotation at Massachusetts General Hospital, Dr. Spencer made a break from psychiatric tradition to reveal herself as a musician. She got permission from her supervisors to organize a concert for the patients on her psychiatric unit. The concert included music by Bach, Handel, Schumann, and Mozart, and the ensemble included musical psychiatrists like herself.

"The concert was fascinating for so many reasons," she recalled. "Some patients have depression with suicidal thoughts. Others experience psychotic symptoms, such as hearing voices that are not real, and some have such severe illness that they are catatonic. Other patients are in various stages of dementia. They didn't all respond to our performance in the same way, of course, but they all seemed to love it.

"There were two patients with severe psychotic illness whose thoughts and actions became a little bit more organized after the performance. While they usually had trouble constructing even a sentence, after the performance they made some quite meaningful and coherent statements.

"There was one patient who had been brought to the hospital malnourished and dehydrated. She had become so paranoid of the outside world, she couldn't leave her house. She would usually rebuke or ignore us, angry that we were holding her in the hospital against her will. She came in, sat, and listened very calmly and quietly, and the next day thanked us and said how beautiful it was. She *thanked us* for our music. I believe that the patients were moved because clinicians were doing something special for them. I think that if other non-medical musicians had come in and played, it would have been meaningful, but in a different way. We were able to expose a side of us they wouldn't otherwise have seen. It was extremely rewarding to everyone involved."

Following the performance, violinist Dr. Justin Chen, another psychiatry resident, was thoughtful. "I've played in small ensembles at healthcare settings before, but today's performances were moving to me in a way I haven't felt before. The experience of performing now for these individuals as a physician as opposed to an undergraduate was deeply powerful. I felt I was touching their lives in a very different but somehow related way."

BALM FOR A BROKEN HEART

A friend of mine discovered that his wife had fallen in love with another man. He wasn't angry so much as he was bewildered and broken and, above all, frightened. Yes, frightened. Because he loved her. Twenty-five years they had been together and he had never fully realized just how much he loved her. He said, "It was like the stars had fallen from the sky."

He was frantic to win back her love, but part of him understood it was beyond his power to repair. She was holding his hand one minute, and the next she was holding another man's hand. And there is nothing you as a doctor can say or do that can suture up that kind of wound. At first he would sit quietly, his mind somewhere else. Then he started having panic attacks. Severe ones. He couldn't focus at work and couldn't sleep. The image of his beloved in another man's arms would rise like a pop-up ad in his head. A psychiatrist prescribed an antidepressant. But those kinds of drugs can only make the lows less low and the highs less high. They couldn't bring back the girl of his dreams.

It took him a long time to come to grips with the fact that she was gone forever. And it took him a longer time to relax and get back into normal life, and sometimes even to laugh. The only thing that helped a little bit was yoga. But he then realized that it wasn't the yoga itself but the *music* the yoga instructor played. He recalls that it was mainly New Age music or Indian music without the harmonic core of Western music. It wandered and repeated and resonated. The instructor told him the music was designed to induce a trancelike calm, to help turn off the "inner dialog" that we all constantly hold with ourselves and cause us to gnaw at our worries like a dog gnaws a bone. For a time, while he was doing his yoga exercises, the music freed him from his endless fretting.

My friend's home and even his workplace were full of memories and associations with his lost wife. There was little escape. But the music became his refuge.

"You Play. You Understand"

Dr. Denise Lotufo, the physical therapist cellist, works in a busy general practice at Harvard University, but in our world she is known to have a special gift in healing fellow musicians. "My number-one priority is to get them back to playing. I've had patients who have had injuries or chronic pain who will put their violin away or will not touch their piano. There's a sense of real loss in these people. You can see that they are desperate to be able play their instrument but they haven't been able to express that to other people, or if they have, they haven't been taken seriously. After all, it's 'only piano,' as some might say to them."

Patients come to her with aching backs or sore shoulders or pain in their elbow or finger joints. Some come through referral from doctors who know she has a special touch with musicians. But many hear of her via word of mouth from fellow musicians. They know she is a skilled therapist, and they know she plays the cello in the LSO.

"They come to me and they say, 'You play. You understand'," she said. "I had a patient the other day who said, 'You speak my language. Do you really think I'll be able to pick up my violin again? I haven't picked it up in years.' I tell them 'I can't guarantee you'll be able to play at the level you played before, but we will get to the point where it will be enjoyable again.' Then as soon as I get patients like that back to playing for five minutes pain-free, there's a joy in their face that is sometimes overwhelming."

Lessons from *El Sistema*

One of the most moving stories I've come across was from my travels in Venezuela, which I touched on earlier in this book.

In 2010 I met Dr. Gonzalo Hidalgo, twenty-five-year-old principal bassoonist of *El Sistema's* most elite orchestra, the Simon Bolivar Youth Orchestra, conducted by Gustavo Dudamel. Dr. Hidalgo had recently graduated from medical school and was about to begin his surgical residency. When I asked him how he was able to attend SBYO's daily evening rehearsals, he explained that almost all of the doctors in the hospital had once been young musicians of *El Sistema* and secretly wished they were still playing in orchestras. He recalls: "There was a time that I was going on tour with the orchestra so I asked my professor if I could take my exams early. He said 'Give me a reason why.' When I told him I was going to perform in Berlin, he changed my schedule.

"*El Sistema* prepares people. It teaches constancy, personal relationships, discipline, and being able to visualize your goals, professionally or personally. A twelve- or thirteen-year-old kid is taught discipline by being in an orchestra. A teenager of that age is not thinking . . . and certainly not thinking about what he wants to be and about being a doctor. But the orchestra teaches discipline. It teaches you how to be in control of yourself. After playing the opening bassoon solo of Stravinsky's *Rite of Spring* to an audience of five thousand people, it is not as scary to give a presentation or to speak with a medical professor! Playing in orchestra gives you control of yourself and confidence, feeling secure in yourself.

"There was a patient in renal failure but she did not want dialysis because she incorrectly thought that dialysis equaled death. She was very depressed. I was doing my psychiatric rotation and was asked to interview her to evaluate how deeply she was depressed. So I started to talk with her and I began to talk about music. She was not a musician. She was very poor. She had not heard of *El Sistema* before, but she had heard of Gustavo Dudamel (conductor of the LA Philharmonic and an *El Sistema* graduate). I could not reason with her that dialysis would help. She was a young woman, with small children, and it did not make sense for her to allow herself to die. I had to try to reach her some other way.

"We started to talk about music at different sessions. I asked her if she had ever heard classical music. She said she had never heard classical music. 'That kind of music is boring. It is music for the rich people.'

"I told her, 'No, not here in Venezuela. Here in Venezuela, music is *not* for the rich people. It is the music for *everyone*. It helps people like you.' I suggested that her son could start an instrument and be a part of *El Sistema*.

"Then I gave her a CD of Tchaikovsky's fifth Symphony. I told her to listen to the second movement of the Tchaikovsky. 'Close your eyes. Think about your life and your kids. Think that you need to live in order to continue to help your children. If you do not live, you will not be there for them, you won't see them grow up, and perhaps see them playing a concert themselves.'

"The next day, I returned to the clinic and her entire family was there. They thanked me and told me that I was a special person who had saved her life. They told me that she had gone home and listened to the CD. She listened to the music and cried and cried. After she listened to the music, she decided she would take the dialysis so she could live for her children.

"I was very touched because it was not a conscious plan for me to give her the CD. I was not expecting this result, but I spoke from my heart because she was depressed and she was behaving as though she had a terminal illness when she really could do something to save herself."

THE SOUNDS OF HEALING

A few years ago, we compiled a CD of excerpts from our concerts, titled "Sounds of Healing" which was distributed to patients and colleagues. When we learned that Senator Edward Kennedy had been diagnosed with a brain tumor, we sent a CD to his office. Much later, a staff member close to the senator shared with us that Kennedy often listened to our music during his many long trips between Cape Cod and Massachusetts General Hospital. To the end, this great man was such a passionate champion of the arts and healthcare in Massachusetts. I can only hope, and believe, that our "Sounds of Healing" helped him a little during his courageous battle with cancer.

So, when choosing a doctor, should you ask, "Where did you go to school? How long have you been practicing medicine?" Certainly. But you might want to add, "What instrument do you play?" Given the high percentage of physicians who are also musicians, you may discover a doctor who might just be a better listener, better collaborator, and better caregiver than you expected—because of music.

PART III

MUSICIAN-PHYSICIANS
AND THE COMMUNITY

From Clashing Chords to Perfect Harmonies

HEALING OUR PATIENTS AND PLAYING our symphonies gives all of us in the Longwood Symphony Orchestra a lot of satisfaction. But, like Bill Kates, the oboe-playing psychiatrist we met earlier, we sometimes feel conflicted about the multiple paths we've chosen. How can he align his identities as physician, musician, family man, and friend?

In the weeks before a concert, Dr. Kates begins his day at 7 A.M., seeing patients, then a break for some exercise, then more patients. After a long and sometimes emotionally draining day, he has a quick dinner and heads off to rehearsal, which can go to 10 P.M. "I am no longer what my mother would call a spring chicken," he said, "I'm really feeling it by the end of rehearsal. I've had some very painful moments. We were rehearsing the Mahler Second Symphony, which has a huge oboe part that kills you no matter what. The conductor wanted to do that at the end of rehearsal at a quarter to ten at night! I was exhausted and trying to play this most beautiful and difficult part. Maestro Noya used to have a pre-concert rehearsal. You'd have to get there early on Saturday night, rehearse for an hour, and then play it over again for the concert. He did the same thing with the Mahler. That stretched me to the limit."

Dr. Kates struggles with many of the same challenges we all share, that come with the profession, including life-or-death emergencies. "I could easily space out in the middle of the rests," he said, "because I'm busy thinking about patients. In the old days I had a lot more worrisome patients. A lot were suicidal. It sometimes got very hard to concentrate and feel calm."

Dr. Kates, who is serious about his Jewish observance, finds himself in conflict about Saturday morning dress rehearsals—rehearsals on his Sabbath day of rest, prayer, and reflection. "I'm not comfortable about it, but I go. Otherwise," he explains, "I couldn't be in the orchestra. So I make some compromises there."

Last year, Bill slipped on the stairs at Boston Latin School, seriously fracturing his elbow. He had to undergo surgery followed by intensive physical therapy which, sadly, kept him out of the orchestra for nearly a year. Now back in the oboe section, Kates looked thoughtful and said, "I have considered retiring. Everyone says, 'Oh, Bill, you'll retire from psychiatry and you'll have more time to play the oboe!' No one understands: You don't retire *into* oboe playing. You retire *from* oboe playing. It requires daily practice, reed-making, and striving to keep my playing up to the demanding standards of this wonderful orchestra. I do think about playing fewer concerts, but playing with such fine and dedicated musicians remains a rich and fulfilling experience. I'm not ready to give that up."

FINDING OUR INNER SELVES

A lot of us are inveterate multitaskers, bordering on workaholics. Well . . . maybe more than "bordering." The idea of doing a lot of disparate things, really well, can be very satisfying. Music has its rewards, but makes a great demand on our time, too. We don't just rehearse for three hours each week. Orchestra-playing requires time to learn the music as individuals, time to practice, and time to learn how our parts fit into the symphony as the composer intended. Finding this time requires a delicate balance, as it can create pressure at work, within our marriages, pressure with our children and friends, and a sense that while we may be living up to our own high standards, it may be coming at a cost to our personal relationships.

PEOPLE I COULD TALK TO

Dr. Wolfram Goessling is a physician specializing in stem cell and cancer research at Brigham and Women's Hospital and the Dana-Farber Institute. He grew up in Germany playing trumpet in church brass ensembles. He speaks earnestly, perhaps a little nervously, and sits forward in his chair to get his point across. Speaking about busy, he has four children and a lab of his own and is well respected in his field of liver cancer. He cares deeply about his medicine and his patients, his family and his music. His short brown hair is always a bit unruly, seems to be going in different directions at once, a little like his frenetic life.

Raised in Germany, Dr. Goessling started out as a neuro-surgical nurse, studied physics in college, then switched fields to study medicine at the University of Witten. Like many of us, his life in music began long before that.

"I've been playing trumpet since I was eight and started the piano at five or six. My mom was an organist and my brother plays the bass. I grew up in the middle of Germany between Hanover and Cologne where they have a rich church brass choir tradition. That movement started at the end of the 1800s. I started in our local church. After a few years, one of my fellow trumpeters said 'you need lessons and I'm going to take you to my teacher,' so I started with the local trumpet teacher in the local orchestra." Ultimately, he found himself studying with the principal trumpet player of the Berlin Philharmonic.

In 1993 he arrived in Boston as a visiting medical student with his girlfriend Helle Sachse (now his wife and another violinist in the LSO), but found himself curiously isolated in his adopted country. There was something missing. It was Helle who saw an ad in the *Boston Phoenix* newspaper announcing that the LSO was seeking a trumpet player, and urged him to audition. He breezed through the audition, which was a triumph, but for Dr. Goessling, the real triumph was finding a place where he felt at home.

"When I came here, I didn't know anybody. These were the first people I could talk to! They spoke my language, the language of music. I had been making music all my life, in my medical school, in my orchestra, and in a local brass sextet. When I came here, I was not only torn away from my family and my classmates in medical school, but all of a sudden there was no way to play trumpet. That was the big thing about Longwood for me . . . that I could play.

"I liked the conductor Francisco Noya a lot. Francisco was . . . maybe loosey-goosey is not the right word. He was very vibrant; he just had a very different style. He liked brass, and I like that, too! Jonathan McPhee was much more 'professional' in terms of what he demanded of the orchestra. Personally, sometimes I think he expected too much of the orchestra because maybe he didn't realize that we all actually have lives in which we already have to perform at a hundred and fifty percent. Everybody in my life—my clinical chief, my research boss, my conductor, my kids . . . —they all expect a lot of me. I'm always performing at the top level every minute, and sometimes that's just not possible.

"We all make choices in life. If I had truly wanted to become a professional trumpet player, I would have done it! I would probably have fallen on my face . . . but sometimes you feel like you permanently have some shortcomings because you can't deliver whatever's expected every minute, and I have to live with that, and that's . . . okay."

One could almost hear the conflicting voices in him as he concluded, "I think Jonathan has a real respect for what we do in our real lives . . . but he expects us to be at the top of our game musically and that's a constant challenge."

PERFORMANCE ANXIETY

Dr. Wright, the bassoonist/internist, said playing in the LSO is "a funny kind of recreation because you put extra pressure on yourself, especially when you are in a group of high achievers like Longwood. If you make a mistake, you let a whole stage full of your colleagues down—not to mention the audience. Every once in a while in a performance I find myself getting tense. Getting ready to do a big solo, I found myself having sleepless nights and cottonmouth. I see that solo coming, I see it coming, I see it coming . . . and soon my heart is ready to jump out of my chest. I think, 'Wasn't this supposed to be fun? Why am I doing this to myself?'

"I am very interested in performance anxiety. I have an actual medical interest in functional gastro-intestinal distur-bances associated with emotion. I've talked with a lot of people at the conservatories who share both their interest and their concerns, particularly with graduate students who often use unprescribed, surreptitious beta-blockers to control perfor-mance anxiety. Some people would say it is the epinephrine that gives the performer that little extra bit of excitement to give a superlative performance, so why would you want to blunt that? But some people find performance anxiety to be crippling and some careers get stopped because people just get overwhelmed. They lose focus and they lose control."

"I still get nervous sometimes," muses Dr. Tom Sheldon. "That was the biggest struggle when I first started playing. In medicine I am a recognized expert. I am well known in the field of radiation oncology and I am well respected. So sud-denly to start playing again where I am not known at all and I've got a long way to go, that was pretty intense. Some of that came from Maestro McPhee, who was always pressuring us to get us to play more professionally. It has taken me years of work to get chill at rehearsals and now to get chill at concerts. But I didn't quit and I actually got better. Now, the ability to sit on that stage and play, and to know that the best I have is indeed good enough, gives me a great feeling."

When the *Wall Street Journal*'s arts critic, Barrymore Scherer, came to Boston in 2005 to get to know the musicians and music of the LSO, he interviewed Dr. Mark C. Gebhardt, clarinetist and Chief of Orthopedics at Beth Israel Deaconess Medical Center. Dr. Gebhardt practices oncologic orthopedics, but is best known in the field for his outstanding work in caring for children with bone cancer, a technically demanding and frequently heart-rending specialty that brings together medical expertise, compassion, and empathy every day. He has also played principal clarinet in the orchestra for twenty-five years, a role that requires him to perform some of the most demanding, and beautiful, solos in the musical literature. He mused, "I used to get very nervous before playing a solo, until I realized, one day, that the worst that could come of a flubbed note or missed entrance would be a few moments' embarrassment. But no one would lose a limb or die. Although I always want to do my best in concert, that thought put it all into perspective."

LAUNDRY ON MY MIND

Making that switch from the examining room or the operating room to the rehearsal hall can be as much of a jolt as it is a comfort. When Maestro Jonathan McPhee first came aboard as conductor, he had to adjust to a very unusual corps of players. I explained to him that professional musicians are usually coming to rehearsal from another rehearsal, a music lesson, or the practice studio. Longwood Symphony members, on the other hand, must often go through a far more radical psychological and sometimes physical transition from doctor to musician, coming from the operating room, intensive care ward, or cancer research laboratory.

"Professional musicians come to rehearsal ready to go from the first bar," McPhee mused. "But the LSO players need at least ten minutes to adjust themselves to the rehearsal situation after dealing all day with life-and-death issues far removed from music." The conductor observed that while professional musicians are trained to respond emotionally from the first downbeat, physicians are trained to avoid personal expression on duty. "So my hardest task in those first ten minutes of rehearsal is to put these players back in touch with their emotions so they can direct them toward the music."

Cellist Denise Lotufo recalls that Jonathan had a hard time with us in the beginning. "He's accustomed to professional musicians. He's used to coming in, giving the downbeat, and—boom—they're on and playing. Our orchestra isn't like that, It takes a little bit of adjustment time. We have day jobs. We come in and we're thinking about a bazillion other things. No matter how good the musicians are in the LSO, they don't have the experience with being 'on' right away with the music. They're used to being 'on' right away in front of that surgery table. I'm 'on' when my patient is telling me the history of what injury they have. Whereas with music it takes a little time to get into it. Rehearsals are at the end of the day, so people are just coming from a heavy day at work.

"I had an interesting and revealing conversation with Jonathan once," she said. "We were talking about how difficult it is to concentrate sometimes through a rehearsal. My mind wanders. I told him I sometimes think about the laundry I have to do at home. And he said, 'You *what*?' I said, 'Don't you ever think about your laundry while you're conducting every now and then?' He just burst out laughing and said, 'NoooOOO.' And I guess that's the difference."

A few summers ago, Dr. Terry Buchmiller, who was performing as concertmaster, called McPhee five minutes before rehearsal was to begin. "I'm closing the final anastomoses [connection] from a small bowel obstruction and will probably be a few minutes late," she apologized. "Can someone else tune the orchestra?"

SILENCE

Although we all love music, there are times when music itself can actually be a stressor versus a stress reliever.

"I like listening to all kinds of music," said Dr. Heidi Kimberly, the emergency room physician/violinist we met in Chapter One. "I grew up with music in a house full of music *and* medicine. My dad is a cardiologist and I always saw that he was very passionate about what he did. Music is a part of who I am. It makes me a happier, more well-rounded, more content person. But I am aware that under certain circumstances, music can also be stressful. It can even get overwhelming, especially in the emergency room. It can be emotionally draining."

Offstage, each of us has a different taste in genres of music, from the grand bombast of some of the great symphonies of the late Romantic period to jazz, pop, and rock. As we move forward, will certain genres of music emerge as more healing or therapeutic for certain patients?

Silence itself can sometimes be its own kind of music. Tamara Goldstein said "There's a quote I really like from Aldous Huxley: 'After silence, that which comes nearest to expressing the inexpressible is music.' All the same, there are some people who thrive in silence. Silence can be healing. Silence is a part of music. It's the space between the notes. As much as music does, for some people turning *off* the music—getting a quiet environment—really helps."

SEEKING HARMONY

As musician-physicians, we will always strive to find the perfect harmonic balance between music and medicine. Like music itself, there is a natural ebb and flow—at a certain time in our careers, medicine will take precedence. Later, music may call. Jazz fusion horn player Eddie Henderson, who I mentioned earlier, earned his medical degree at Howard University and practiced medicine for a decade before finally returning full-time to music. Even after the lucky break that launched him into a big-time career, Dr. Henderson continued to practice psychiatry for a time.[1]

Some of the best musician-physicians go all the way through medical school, but then decide that the pull of music is too strong. England's Sir Jeffrey Tate, inspired by the caring and devotion his surgeons demonstrated in caring for his congenital spina bifida, went on to medical school and became a practicing eye surgeon for a time at St. Thomas's Hospital in London. But his main love was opera, and he eventually left medicine altogether to become one of the operatic world's most respected conductors.

Uruguayan-born musician and composer Jorge Drexler was the first from his country to win an Oscar (in 2004 for

"Al Otro Lado del Río" from the film *The Motorcycle Diaries*). He earned a degree as an otolaryngologist (ear, nose, and throat doctor) from La Universidad de la República Oriental del Uruguay in 1992. But in that same year he released the first of more than a dozen albums, eventually becoming an international star in South America, Europe, and the United States with a distinctive mix of jazz, pop, and the music of his homeland. Although he came from a family of doctors, he never practiced.[2]

Dr. Lakshminarayana Subramaniam is master of musical fusion of the classical styles of India and the West. A child-prodigy violinist and composer, he graduated from Madras Medical College but never actually practiced, turning almost immediately back to his childhood fascination with music and launching a major writing, recording, and performing career that included pieces for movies, ballets, and classical orchestras.

And then there is the unusual case of another ophthalmologist, the brilliant conductor Dr. Sam Wong (no relation), who made a long round trip from medicine to music and back again. Born in Hong Kong, he began studying piano at an age when most kids start learning the alphabet. His family moved to Toronto when he was nine and he enrolled in the Royal Conservatory of Music. At Harvard, rather than music or medicine, he majored in applied mathematics and developed his conducting chops as leader of Harvard's student-run Bach Society Orchestra. His Chinese parents discouraged him from music, and encouraged him to follow a more stable path in medicine, so he went on to Harvard Medical School, during which time the Longwood Symphony Orchestra invited him to conduct a summer concert. Wong eventually interrupted his training as an ophthalmologist at the New York Eye and Ear Institute when he was tapped to be the music director of the New York Youth Symphony in Carnegie Hall and the assistant conductor of the New York Philharmonic under Leonard Bernstein. He spent the next twenty years conducting around the world, including Hong Kong and Honolulu, but medicine was never far away.

Wong finally finished his ophthalmology training a few years ago and is now back in New York practicing as an ophthalmologist and has also founded the Global Music Healing Institute. Like the musicians of the Longwood Symphony Orchestra, Dr. Wong is organizing symposia that explore the delicate intersection between the healing arts of music and medicine. Describing the tension between his two careers, he told us, "It's like riding two horses growing apart, being drawn and halved," he told us. "Those strong feelings are always tugging."

GREAT EXPECTATIONS

Even our youngest and most energetic members experience some of these conflicts—music versus medicine, guilt, jealousy, politics, trying to balance their own lives, seeking what affects their spirits. How they get along with one another. How they get along with the conductor. How they deal with patients' expectations when patients place their lives in our trust. On one hand, TV medical dramas have raised people's expectations to an unrealistic height. On the other hand, we're acutely aware that some of the bad apples in our profession have lowered people's regard for us. They find some of us imperious, detached, egotistical, poor listeners, and even sloppy.

And medicine is confronting larger conflicts as an institution. Coping with the high cost of medical care has prompted a national dialogue—some would say a battle—over how health care will be financed in twenty-first-century America. Those questions weigh on us as doctors. We look to our music as a refuge, but even there, change is coming. Many of our older members recall a time when the LSO was as much a social group as a musical group. It was a low-pressure place for music lovers to get together and have fun playing music they loved without worrying about being technically perfect. This pleasant atmosphere ironically brought about its own end. The music and the mission attracted more applicants. More applicants meant more competition. More competition led to a sharp increase in the quality and motivation of our new members. The increasing quality raised expectations among both the players and the audiences. Our members still love what they do, and the LSO of 2012 is a much tighter and more professional organization than the LSO of 1991. But have the raised expectations altered the atmosphere and made it a little bit more like work?

This syndrome has also created something of a generation gap within the orchestra. We have some older members whose musical skills may not match up to some of the younger members. But there is a substantial bloc in the orchestra that believes that's perfectly Okay. All ages still share a love of playing this great music. And there is great warmth between players of all generations. Interestingly, all of us have technically improved over the years. Many of us have been motivated to buy new instruments and to resume our music lessons. And just as some older physicians demonstrate the best clinical skills, some of the old guard have the best "orchestra sense," that ability to hear across the ensemble, to collaborate closely with a stand partner and to anticipate a conductor's tempo. A seat in the LSO is not a lifetime appointment. With very few exceptions, members make their own decisions about when it's time for them to retire.

I don't think this whole process is unique to the LSO by any means. Many organizations go through this same evolution, as the founders hand off to a new generation with a slightly different interpretation of the group's mission. As the years go by and the LSO continues to attract younger members even as it gets older, I'll be interested to see how this marvelous organism evolves.

ALL TOGETHER NOW

So, how to reconcile the forces that threaten to pull us apart? Our medical careers versus our musical careers? Work versus family? Informal versus formal? Old versus young? I think it all comes back to the music. If we use music to heal our patients and ourselves, we should use music to heal the divides within the LSO.

Denise Lotufo said, "The beauty of the LSO is that everybody in that audience loves you, regardless. Our audience believes in what we do. I don't think we'd have the audience if they didn't. They'd love us whether we play the right notes or not. There is an energy that comes across whether it's during the moments when they're applauding and even when they're just listening. You can feel it. It's like electricity. And we get standing ovations quite often, and bravos now and then, which is nice. And in those moments it's possible to forget anything that may be bothering us or dividing us."

13

Bringing the Humanities Back to Medicine

The Longwood Symphony has made a difference in the lives of countless individuals
and, in doing so, has inspired others to
follow its lead."
—Senator Edward M. Kennedy, 2007

THROUGHOUT THIS BOOK I HAVE described how the LSO is
using its medical and musical expertise in a unique way—we
call it "Healing our Community through Music." This has
been the orchestra's guiding principle through my twenty
years with the organization. It is a carefully thought-out
strategy that I believe is worth emulating by arts groups and
medical/science groups everywhere.

Michael Barnett joined the LSO Board of Directors a few years ago as a student representative and immediately embraced his role with conviction and energy. Over the past two years, he has served as Chair of the Community Engagement Committee, playing a key role in identifying the healthcare nonprofits we collaborate with during the concert season, through our LSO Healing Art of Music program.

"It's really important to me," he said. "It combines our music and medicine aspects, and tells the world that we feel, as doctors, that it is really important for us to give back and to improve the health of our communities. We are lucky to put on these amazing concerts and play amazing music. Then we structure them so that each concert promotes, not only ourselves, but also promotes someone in our community who is doing really great work."

There is a traditional Chinese proverb that I've always tried to live by: *Give a man a fish and you feed him for a day. Teach a man to fish and you feed him for a lifetime.* Whether it is helping a young medical student come up with the right diagnosis or helping a young musician understand a piece of music, or working with a patient coping with an illness, this proverb has always rung true. Instead of treating only the immediate symptoms, trying to help a patient or parent change lifestyle habits ultimately leads to a healthier family. If I help a medical student think through the disease process rather than telling her the diagnosis, she will remember the case. Similarly with the Longwood Symphony: instead of simply playing a benefit performance for a healthcare organization, which may be helpful in the short run, working with them to create an event for themselves does more to help it promote its stature in the community, and sometimes its organizational structure.

A concert with our Community Partners is a true collaboration—together we are learning to fish. Through the purchase of a block of deeply discounted tickets and an investment of staff and volunteer time, each organization becomes a *collaborator* rather than a *beneficiary*. Each Community Partner creates its own special event around our concerts and, with close and constant guidance by LSO volunteers and staff over many months, the organization learns important lessons in marketing, messaging, and fundraising. We encourage our Community Partners to use the concert to tell their story, from focusing on public health challenges for women in the developing world (Physicians for Human Rights), to honoring the physicians who care for children with neurodegenerative diseases (Familes of SMA), to reminding the public about the ongoing medical challenges that patients faced from radiation exposure (Children of Chernobyl). The organizations are encouraged to bring their staff, patients, and families to be part of the concert as well, to share in the musical healing.

Michael Barnett articulates this well: "We try to create a relationship between us and them. We promote them in our mailings and on our website, and they promote us to their benefactors and their beneficiaries. We've been doing this for nearly twenty years, and the list of charities seeking to partner with us gets longer each year as our reputation grows.

"Each concert event is different—and unique to the organization we are benefitting. For example, for our concert with The Food Project (which teaches urban farming and nutrition to inner-city kids in Boston), we sent chamber music groups to perform at several of their hunger relief organizations—to give them a dose of musical therapy, and maybe attract a few more attendees as well. We're constantly trying to come up with creative ways to build a foundation, a relationship with the other organization that will last for years. I still get people who come up to me and say: 'I heard you had a concert for The Food Project. I wish I could have been there.' That is real success to me, because it shows we created some buzz in the community, that otherwise wouldn't necessarily have had this organization on its radar."

To date, the LSO has partnered with close to forty non-profit health organizations in our community since 1991. Nearly all of the organizations continue to grow and thrive in Boston, and we've maintained a relationship with most of the organizations we have partnered with over the years. With some organizations, such as the Albert Schweitzer Fellowship and Boston's Healthcare for the Homeless Program, it has been a twenty-year journey together.

In 2007, the Longwood Symphony was recognized as a national model, receiving the MetLife Excellence in Community Engagement Award from the League of American Orchestras, which wrote, "When an arts organization makes itself so indispensable to the well-being of a community, it not only helps the long-term health of that community, the organization also helps ensure its own survival."

A few stories will illustrate how valuable these programs have become to our community, and to the LSO.

SAVING A LIFE AND RESTORING A FAMILY

On a Saturday summer afternoon in 1989, a young man came to my office. He was the last patient of the day. He was of Korean descent, having been adopted as a young child by an American family in Norwell, Massachusetts. There were two Caucasian biological sisters and two adopted Korean children in the family.

Jonathan McGowan had just graduated from Norwell High School and was eager to pursue his business degree at the prestigious Babson College in the fall. He was taking a summer tennis program at a local college but came to me, puzzled by the development of multiple bruises on his legs and arms. "Did you fall on the court?" I asked him. "Did you hit yourself with the racket?" He had not. I drew some lab tests and sent him home, only to call him back right away. The blood smear was abnormal; the diagnosis was leukemia.

Rather than entering Babson College that fall, Jonathan entered Children's Hospital of Boston, where he spent the majority of his next two years.

Over the past decades, the cure rate for childhood leukemia has steadily risen. Chemotherapy courses have been refined to reduce long-term toxicity. Still, there are some forms of the disease that are more virulent than others. Unfortunately, Jonathan had a particularly aggressive illness; he suffered two relapses and it seemed that his cancer was becoming progressively more resistant to the chemotherapeutic agents offered. His oncologists determined that Jonathan would need a bone marrow transplant to survive.

Like a fingerprint, everyone has a unique set of HLA markers. In order to minimize the chance for rejection, doctors try to find a donor whose HLA sequence (human leukocyte antigen) is most similar to that of the patient. Sadly, at that time in the late '80s, the national Bone Marrow Donor Registry had only three thousand donors of Asian ancestry in their files, and none were close enough matches to be suitable for Jonathan.

Ever resourceful, and desperate to find a solution to save their son, the McGowan family reached out to the adoption agency that had first introduced them to Jonathan. They learned that Jonathan's biologic brother had been adopted by a family in Switzerland. Now twenty-two years old, this young man agreed to come to the United States to be tested and to see his younger brother again. Sadly, what must have been a happy reunion on many levels was bittersweet; his brother's bone marrow was not a close enough match.

At the same time, Jonathan's adoptive sisters, both in college, were organizing bone marrow drives on college campuses across the country. They needed money for travel and supplies.

That is when Longwood Symphony agreed to dedicate its next concert to raising funds for the National Marrow Donor Program. In this case, while we did not raise a large amount of money, our concert brought together students from many of Boston's colleges, and raised awareness in the community about the National Bone Marrow Registry. It garnered the gratitude of the nurses and doctors at Children's Hospital caring for so many leukemia patients like Jonathan who were waiting for The Match. The concert enabled Jonathan's sisters to organize five more bone marrow drives on college campuses and spread the word to other students across the country. Through our efforts and those of many others in the community, they grew the Asian bone marrow registry numbers from the initial 3,000 to over 11,000! While none of these 8,000 new donors turned out to be a match for Jonathan, I can't help but think of the hundreds of other patients over the years who *did* find a match from the Bone Marrow Registry, not knowing that the registry had been expanded by the generous act by these young people twenty years ago.

The wonderful epilogue to this story is that Jonathan eventually did find a match: his own biological mother in Korea. The adoption agency that had so lovingly found a family for Jonathan fifteen years before had kept such good records that they were able to locate her and reunite her with her dying son. A few months later, she gave him life for a second time, through a successful bone marrow transplant. A deep and lasting relationship has developed now among the son who has been cured of his cancer, his biological Korean mother, and his adoptive American mother.

EXPRESSING CHILDHOOD TRAUMA THROUGH THE ARTS: BERKSHIRE CHILDREN AND FAMILIES

In June 2010, the Longwood Symphony made its debut at Seiji Ozawa Hall on the famous Tanglewood grounds in Lenox, Massachusetts. This beautiful thousand-seat concert hall was designed by architect William Rawn to look like a Japanese jewel box. The acoustics rival any fine concert hall in the world, including our home base, Jordan Hall.

Our LSO Community Partner in June was Berkshire Children and Families of Massachusetts (BCFMA), a nonprofit organization dedicated to the education and health promotion of impoverished women and children in Pittsfield, Massachusetts and the surrounding communities.

We worked with BCFMA to identify a goal for the weekend's activities. They wanted to raise awareness about domestic violence and its impact on children, and discuss ways the community could work together at prevention, including the use of the arts and increasing childhood and maternal literacy. On the day prior to the concert, Berkshire Children and Families invited educators, social workers, foster parents, and leaders from other local social service agencies to come together for a conference they called "Focus on Families." It was the first time many of these dedicated individuals had a chance to meet each other in their own community. Encouraging BCFMA to utilize the arts to express some of the hard issues they were tackling and to incorporate music as a metaphor for family discord and healing, we opened the day with a presentation and performance by a specially chosen quartet from the Longwood Symphony. Pediatric surgeon and violinist Dr. Terry Buchmiller shared her challenges in the emergency room as the first response caregiver for young trauma victims of child abuse. I discussed the long-term role of a pediatrician who cares for fractured families. Violist Dr. Andrea Spencer discussed her research using child-friendly techniques to elicit responses from neglected children living in poverty in Colombia. And psychologist cellist Dr. Tai Katzenstein introduced the audience to a new evaluation and treatment program being developed at Massachusetts General Hospital to help violent children modify their behavior. Following our discussion, we performed the first movement of Mozart's String Quartet in C major, nicknamed "Dissonant" for the haunting and disturbing suspended chords that open the piece. We presented the work to the audience as a metaphor for a family in crisis—following the ominous introduction, the quartet bursts into a sunny exposition of the hopeful rising themes in C major, Mozart's happiest key. This is soon followed by a dark development section in which the rising themes are splintered, more questioning and doubtful. Finally, the recapitulation, a final resolution with return of themes, initially in the key of G major but finally settling back in the home key of C major. The hopeful theme returns, but is this time expressed by different voices, analogous to a healed family finding its new inner strengths.

Later in the conference, which also included riveting talks by Dr. Carolyn Burns, BCFMA's executive director, and others, we were joined by Dr. Eli Newberger, an emeritus professor at Harvard Medical School and national expert on child abuse. Dr. Newberger is also one of New England's most-renowned tuba players, who performed in Boston's New Black Eagle Jazz Band, an ensemble which he founded, for over thirty years. At this conference he was called upon for his expertise in child abuse and also as a keyboardist/ conductor of a small ensemble arrangement of "Tubby the Tuba." This musical tale, written in 1945 by Paul Tripp, was perhaps better known to a previous generation. I remember listening to it often as a child, when my mother played the

LP for us as we lay down for our naps. It is a perfect parable about the ostracized child: *Tubby the Tuba is a member of the brass section in an orchestra conducted by the great Senor Pizzicato. Poor Tubby is relegated to the bass line in the orchestra, sadly playing his "oompah oompah" while the fiddles, flutes and other instruments dance merrily through the musical scale. When he's tried to express his dissatisfaction, he is derided by the other more melodic instruments. One day, Tubby meets a bullfrog who teaches him a beautiful melody and asserts that Tubby, too, should have a voice in the group. The next day, Tubby eagerly returns to the orchestra, armed with his new Tune, only to find himself ridiculed once more by all the other instruments. Finally, encouraged by the conductor and his only friend, Pico the Piccolo, Tubby shyly introduces his Tune. The orchestra is enchanted, and the piece ends with all forces happily playing the Tune together in harmony, fortissimo!*

The conference was a huge success—it raised community awareness about Berkshire Children and Families that resulted in new referrals and new lines of communication between caregivers in the Pittsfield community. The next evening, many came to Ozawa Hall to hear the Longwood Symphony's performance of Debussy, Nielsen, and a commissioned work by Gene Scheer about the life of Dr. Albert Schweitzer. Later, the leadership of Berkshire Children and Families gathered and we brainstormed about how BCFMA could continue to incorporate music into its work. Inspired by the LSO's performance and the discussions that followed, and thanks to the vision of its Board and Executive Director, Carolyn Burns, the decision was made to launch the first-ever *El Sistema*-inspired program for at-risk children of Pittsfield in the fall of 2011, under the name Music 4 Children.

BUILDING A DREAM:
MATTAPAN COMMUNITY HEALTH CENTER

Some of our Community Partners tackle big challenges and come up with even bigger solutions. One such organization is the Mattapan Community Health Center (MCHC), led by the dynamic and irrepressible Dr. Azzie Young, its CEO and president. MCHC provides healthcare for one of Boston's poorest communities, which suffers from some of the city's most serious health problems, with high rates of prematurity and low-birth-weight infants; increased mortality due to heart disease and lung cancer; high rates of HIV/AIDS; and more deaths by homicide. MCHC has been working out of a small, cramped health clinic on Blue Hill Avenue since 1972, remarkably serving more than seven thousand patients each year in that tiny facility. But despite its suboptimal physical space, once you enter the crowded waiting room, you feel a sense of safety, warmth, and caring—this is a healing space, one that treats over 7,000 patients a year.

A leader in public health, Azzie Young, Ph.D., M.S., M.P.A., has seen much in her twenty-five years in public health administration. Yet she remains positive and upbeat and advocates tirelessly for her mainly Latino and Haitian patient population. Rather than dwell on the adversities faced in the Mattapan community, she treasures the successes. One story with a happy ending is about a 79-year-old indigent patient who presented with dysphagia, or difficulty swallowing food, which progressed to a difficulty swallowing liquids. Tests at the Boston Medical Center revealed a cancer of the esophagus. He had chemotherapy, surgery, and radiation, and, as of this writing, has done very well. Dr. Young relates that, at MCHC, all patients receive thoughtful, respectful care, with no consideration of age, ethnicity, or financial status.

When I met with Dr. Young and members of MCHC's board and staff in the fall of 2004, I asked our standard, open-ended question, "What do you hope to accomplish with your concert with Longwood Symphony?" The answer was unambiguous and ambitious. "We want to use our concert to launch a campaign for a new health care facility in their neighborhood." The community, they reasoned, deserved far better than their current space could offer, and with a new facility, they could expand their preventive health programs, especially for women and children.

They understood that this concert could be an opportunity to gather civic and business leaders together with members of Boston's healthcare community. The concert of Mozart, Hindemith, and Wagner was held on October 7, 2005. It raised over $30,000 and publicly launched their capital building campaign.

In 2010 Mattapan Community Health Center honored the Longwood Symphony with its Community Health Pinnacle Award, which I accepted on behalf of the orchestra. The award was given for "outstanding support of community health centers and in healing our communities through music." We consider this to be among our proudest honors.

Five years later, Dr. Azzie Young is realizing the dream and vision she had for the patients of her community. On September 10, 2010 she was joined by Massachusetts Governor Deval Patrick and Boston Mayor Tom Menino, to break ground on a new community and women's health clinic in the heart of Mattapan. It is scheduled to open in the spring of 2012.

HEALING IN THE FAMILY: AMERICAN EPILEPSY SOCIETY

Some of our stories are even closer to home. Dr. Susan Spencer was a national leader in the field of epilepsy and the Chair of Neurology at Yale Medical School. She was also a musician-physician who played piano and flute. With her husband, Dr. Dennis Spencer, Yale's Chair of Neurosurgery, they had twin musician-physician daughters, Andrea and Joanna. Andrea joined the LSO when she was a first-year medical student and has played with the orchestra throughout her medical school training, internship, and residency. Sadly, Dr. Susan Spencer died unexpectedly two years ago. Andrea, still a resident doctor in training, was devastated. Knowing how much the Longwood Symphony had meant to the entire Spencer family, we found a way for LSO's Healing Art of Music program to honor and memorialize Susan Spencer. The 2009 Annual Meeting of the American Epilepsy Society (AES), an organization in which Susan Spencer had been integrally involved, was being held in Boston for the first time in many years. Since the conference coincided exactly with the LSO's December concert, we invited the members of American Epilepsy Society to attend. It made sense for us to dedicate our first concert to Dr. Spencer's memory and to use the concert to launch a new research fund in her name. The concert drew nearly nine hundred people, including three hundred and twenty-five neurologists from across the country.

The music was profoundly fitting for the evening. Although the repertoire had been chosen more than a year earlier, it seemed as though it had been selected for just this occasion. The LSO performed the New England premiere of *STYX*, a work by Giya Kancheli for mixed chorus, large orchestra, and viola solo. Violist Roger Tapping and the New World Chorale joined the Longwood Symphony for this moving and dramatic work. Written in memory of some of his dearest friends, Kancheli created a piece that depicted the journey of Charon, the mythical Greek boatman who ferried souls between the land of the living and the dead, across the river Styx. Like Dr. Andrea Spencer herself, the voice that spoke across the chasm of life and death was expressed through the viola. There is a clear parallel between Charon's role and that of our own as physicians and musicians. As healers and comforters, we are both privileged and challenged to serve to journey with our patients and audiences to the shores between life and death.

"We had a full house that night," Spencer recalled. "I'll never forget sitting in Jordan Hall, filled with people who knew my mother and loved her and listening to this orchestra supporting her. It was an amazing night for me and spoke to the role the orchestra has come to play in my life and in my family's life. I'm so lucky to have that kind of support network."

LSO ON CALL

As previously mentioned, LSO on Call is our musical equivalent of an ambulance service. Small ensembles of two or three musicians bring music to nursing homes, hospitals, and homeless shelters on a monthly basis. This is bringing music to the bedside—an intense experience for musician and patient alike.

"Playing for patients is totally different from playing for a regular audience," said Sherman Jia, LSO concertmaster and

Harvard Medical student. Jia is as serious a musician as he is a medical student and takes part regularly in LSO on Call. "Patients are actually a lot more responsive and appreciative. This is especially true for elderly patients who are in nursing homes for a long time. A lot of times they don't get as much interaction with people from the outside—or even from their doctors—as they really deserve. It's very rewarding to go as a musician and a physician and interact with patients at that level. When you arrive at a health care facility to play, you see a lot of patients sitting there in their wheelchairs. They see all these strangers with instruments and they don't know what to expect. Most of them don't really listen to classical music. For a lot of them, to see classical music played live, sometimes for the first time, it's really different for them, and it's really engaging. A lot of people go from a state of being tired, lethargic, and not really with-it to all of a sudden really excited and really happy. You can see patients tapping their feet, or humming, or getting up and dancing sometimes. Often it's as simple as seeing a patient's face light up."

LONDON BOUND—AND BEYOND?

One of the long-term dreams of the Longwood Symphony Orchestra's members has been to share its model internationally through medical/musical tours. In June 2008, a contingent of thirty-five members of the LSO partnered with colleagues in London on just such a tour. The concerts and lectures were given to benefit Marie Curie Cancer Care, the largest hospice program in the U.K. "It was one of the best moments any of us has ever had," recalled surgeon/violist Dr. Nicholas Tawa. "Music, community service, and the educational part—the London trip showed how we could really put it all together." A small planning group traveled to London in January to meet with physicians, hospice coordinators, and concert planners to set the itinerary. The trip took over a year to plan and was paid for through individual fundraising and benefit chamber music performances.

Conductor Jonathan McPhee, an American conductor who spent many of his formative years in London at the Royal Academy of Music, chose a program that was a balance of British and American composers and perfectly suited for our small ensemble of thirty-five musicians. Highlights included Ralph Vaughan Williams' *Lark Ascending,* performed by British violinist David Juritz, and Samuel Barber's *Knoxville Summer of 1914,* performed by American soprano Janna Baty. The concert culminated with Aaron Copland's signature work, *Appalachian Spring.* For McPhee, this work was a homecoming for him; as a young man, he had worked with American choreographer Martha Graham, and had conducted *Appalachian Spring* in London with her dance company.

Our own tour opened with a six-hour conference on "Innovations in Cancer Care" at St. Bartholomew's Hospital, London's oldest hospital, which was founded in 1123. Under the watchful eye of the hospital's later champion, King Henry VIII, LSO members shared knowledge with their British oncology counterparts, discussing new techniques in medical and surgical intervention, new findings in cancer research, and new perspectives on cancer prevention. In the afternoon, some of us toured the hospital's recently refurbished bone marrow transplant unit. Finally, we changed into concert dress, rearranged the chairs in the Great Hall, took out our instruments, and performed a concert to raise funds for the new facility.

The rest of the week proceeded in much the same way. There were morning meetings with medical colleagues and afternoon chamber music for patients and evening performances for larger audiences. Each member had a slightly different agenda, according to their interests and areas of expertise. Senior cancer biologist cellist Dr. Heidi Greulich traveled to Oxford to give a lecture on molecular biology, while palliative care nurse cellist Nancy Chane traveled to Syndenham to St. Christopher's Hospice where the hospice movement was founded by Dame Cicely Saunders in 1967. At St. Christopher's we met a music therapist, Nigel Hartley, a professionally trained pianist. Years ago, he found it more rewarding to share music with his patients in hospice than on the concert stage and since then had become a prominent music therapist, authoring *The Creative Arts in Palliative Care*.

"Funny things always happen with this orchestra," mused Dr. Tawa. He recalled how one of our London concerts was delayed—by the Queen! Her Majesty was across the street celebrating the four hundredth anniversary of the Temple Church and all roads were blocked off for security. As her motorcade passed, she waved to our astonished musicians, and soon the audience arrived and the performance began.

"THERE'S MORE," TAWA WENT ON. "We were getting ready to give our biggest performance and we were playing *Appalachian Spring* by Copland that night. In the afternoon, though, we took a sightseeing tour to Windsor Castle. A British military band came out for the Changing of the Guard, and they began to play 'Simple Gifts,' the Shaker melody that forms the basis for that piece! And it was absolutely bizarre that a British military orchestra would be playing an American hymn tune two hours before we were going to give our performance. Funny things like that occur.

"On the final day," continued Tawa, "we went to St. Paul's Cathedral to attend the service and to hear a performance of the Vaughan Williams 'Mass in g minor.' The vicar gives this sermon on how Life is about taking risks. Here, we were in the middle of a trip that almost didn't come off because some people balked at the last minute, and it was just like God speaking to us and telling us that we had done the right thing."

I remember that day. We were all profoundly moved by the service. Afterward, I went up to the pastor to thank him and told him about the orchestra, that we were an orchestra of healthcare providers who had just spent a week raising money for cancer, meeting with cancer specialists, and playing for patients in hospice. He replied, "I felt a strong sense of healing in the church today and I didn't know why until now."

One of the most moving stories from our trip to London is from Dr. Mark C. Gebhardt, chief of orthopedics at Beth Israel Deaconess Hospital and clarinetist. While he is also a general orthopedist, Gebhardt has the specialty of caring for children with bone cancer, or osteosarcoma. "About a year ago I met a little girl from Puerto Rico who had a malignant bone tumor of her tibia. She was sent to me to excise her tumor after some extensive preoperative chemotherapy. Because she was only seven years old at the time, the removal of the tumor below her knee would leave her with a major inequality of the lengths of her legs. Fortunately, there are internal metal prostheses that can replace certain bones (in this case the tibia) and can be 'expanded' or lengthened in small increments as the child grows. The expectation is that by the end of growth, the two limbs will be equal length. One of the pioneers in this field of prosthesis manufacture and scientific development is a biomechanics laboratory at the Royal National Orthopaedic Hospital in London. The Centre for Biomedical Engineering has become Stanmore Implants Worldwide Ltd., a company that has a specific interest in making custom prostheses for limb salvage following tumor resections. I had them make one for my little patient and it has so far worked beautifully.

"While in London, I visited with the bioengineers and technicians at Stanmore to plan the first lengthening for my little patient. It was a morning well spent. I got to tour the facility and see first-hand how they computer-model the implants and physically make them. I got a demonstration about how the expansion works and planned a trip for them to come to Boston for the first expansion. This is truly an innovative group that maintains a close tie to the University and they are clearly leaders in the field of tumor prostheses. In addition to enhancing the scientific collaborations, they kindly donated funds to the London tour that sponsored a medical student for the trip.

"The emotion of my work and living with life and death and limbs—about preserving-or-not situations—gives me a certain pathos that comes out in the music. I think in some way the fact that I'm a musician makes it possible for me to deal with these people and these cases . . . a lot of people could not do what I do. The music sort of helps that, but it's tough to draw a straight line connecting the two."

Gebhardt went on, "Physicians as a group, and especially surgeons, are probably in the top one percent of income in this country. And that puts the onus on us to give back. 'To those whom much is given, much is expected.' And while I originally joined the LSO for the purely selfish motivation that I wanted to play music, now I think it's great that we have raised so much for so many good causes."

LSO's Healing Art of Music program has been a way to use music to help the community. We at the LSO want to use our music as a voice beyond entertainment or just making someone feel good. We know innately that music can strike even deeper than that. In conservatories, music students are now given opportunities, not only to play on concert hall stages, but to play at homeless shelters, in schools, and even in hospitals. This is an encouraging sign for the future of music. In 2010, after the devastating earthquake in Haiti, students from every music school in Boston and two professional ensembles joined the LSO on stage to raise funds for Partners in Health in a concert *Symphonic Relief for Haiti*. Just two weeks after the earthquake, two hundred musicians gathered on the Jordan Hall stage to raise nearly $100,000 for earthquake relief.

And there's another dividend from our charitable work, an artistic one. When people are playing beyond themselves, the music simply gets better.

What's next? Tawa mused, "It would probably be even more meaningful if we could go to a non–First World environment—notably Albert Schweitzer's Africa, but that gets really tricky. You have to have an infrastructure that can receive you and really benefit from it. So you have to have physicians there who are sophisticated enough to benefit from what we have to teach. You have to have a government that is not going to exploit you for their own purposes, you have to have an audience that is not just the elites of that Third World country, but the actual people. So going from Europe to Africa would be a big leap."

That's among the open vistas that await the organization—and others like it. Combining music, medicine, and service is never easy, which doesn't mean we can't strive for it. We have something special to contribute: our willingness to volunteer our time and skills to help those who need help the most. We love to play in this kind of harmony with our community.

14

Tomorrow's Musician-Physicians

IN 1993 AT THE BETH Israel Deaconess Medical Center, a baby was born. His life outside the womb began more than three months ahead of schedule.

He was a miracle. Weighing only twenty-two ounces at birth, he spent the first few months of his life in an incubator, listening to the rhythm of his respirator and the beeps of his heart monitor, with his concerned parents hovering over him. It takes an entire dedicated medical village to help a young premature infant successfully navigate his way from the delivery room to the Newborn Intensive Care Unit (NICU) and finally home to his family. Doctors, nurses, respiratory therapists, and specialized dieticians work together as a symphony of caregivers, with the occasional soloist ophthalmologist, cardiologist, or neurologist dropping by to add their expertise and advice.

This amazing baby overcame most of the obstacles arrayed against him and finally went home with his parents around his original due date. By then he weighed nearly four pounds, and had a whole community behind him, cheering him on. An ongoing miracle.

Up to this point, the baby could have been any child. The love and care that he received from the dedicated team is extended to every baby in every NICU, and the hope for each one to succeed is uniform. There is no greater joy among the members of the team than to see a baby successfully discharged from their care.

But this particular child, whose name is Jeremiah Klarman, was a special child. Who knows how the early rhythms of the NICU impacted his sense of patterns? Of sound? His family members remember that he was always a musical child, even as a toddler. Jeremiah wrote his first piece of music at age five and was playing piano sonatas by age seven. His piano teacher, mentor, and coach, Angel Rivera, recalls, "He was so full of music and so full of musical ideas, it was constantly flowing out of him. My job was to help him control the flow, without suppressing his enthusiasm."

Through the early years, Rivera carefully guided Jeremiah's musical training on the piano, taught him about composition, and even recommended a violin teacher for him when the young prodigy wanted to start another instrument. And when it became clear that Jeremiah was destined to be a composer, Rivera introduced him to Rodney Lister, a master composer and composition teacher at the New England Conservatory with a special talent for mentoring young composers. I met Jeremiah when he was twelve years old at his end-of-year recital, which he performed with a group of talented young musical friends. His works included piano pieces, string quartets, and piano quartets. Lister later told me that Jeremiah was so prolific that, had they not limited the repertoire, the concert would have gone on for two more hours.

Training a young composer is a very special apprenticeship. Under Lister's tutelage, the young man explored the musical literature of the past, composing various works "in the style of" the great masters. This careful training technique is a tradition that has been passed on through the ages: Mozart and Beethoven had similar training. In the visual art world, Picasso's early paintings, too, look to the art of the past. In order to develop his own style, he first had to master the styles of others. But even though many of Klarman's early works were held within these musical parameters, one could always hear his distinct voice in the music, full of humor, thoughtful introspection, and sometimes profound sentiment.

A MUSICAL VILLAGE

A new village now embraced him—a musical village. The youth orchestras at the New England Conservatory premiered his symphonies. His synagogue sang his choral works. His music camp played his chamber music. Finally, even the Boston Pops featured one of his symphonic compositions on "From the Top," a National Public Radio broadcast that showcases brilliant young talent.

The Longwood Symphony Orchestra, too, developed a long-running special relationship with Jeremiah Klarman. We have championed his works for several years. In 2008, Jeremiah's *Festive Dance* was performed at the LSO's annual free summer concert to an appreciative crowd of eight thousand people at the Hatch Shell on the Esplanade. Later that season, he was invited by conductor Jonathan McPhee into the orchestra pit of Boston Ballet to observe a rehearsal. There he sat in rapt silence, following the entire three-hour *Romeo and Juliet* score, then inquiring about a few note discrepancies in the violin section. His future is bright. Eighteen years old in 2011, he will be a composition major and continue his piano studies at the New England Conservatory of Music.

Late in 2010, McPhee announced that he would be stepping down from the LSO podium to pursue other musical commitments. When he took his final bow on March 19, 2011, ending six years of fine musical leadership, the Longwood Symphony Orchestra surprised him with a high musical honor—a commissioned brass fanfare, *McPhee's Magic,* written by Klarman and dedicated to the Maestro. As we search for the new music director who will chart the next part of our musical journey, I know that Klarman's music, and the music of other promising young talent, will continue to be featured in our performances in the future, in addition to our continued benefit work for the medical community and those in need.

I've told Klarman's story because my Longwood Symphony Orchestra has lived a life very much the same as his. Music and medicine have intertwined in both from their earliest days, both proved to be prodigies who benefitted from a series of enlightened stewards, and both have been incalculably enriched by their experiences. And now here's the key connection. I believe both Klarman and the LSO are dynamic youngsters on the threshold of a bright future. What will that future look like?

To find out, I sought out the opinions of my fellow LSO musicians and asked each of them to gaze into their personal crystal ball and tell me what they saw.

The Seven Ages of the LSO

Denise Lotufo, the cellist and physical therapist, compared the life of the LSO over the past three decades to the life of a person. "We went through all the stages. At the beginning we were like a child. We grew like a child with our conductors as parents. We took on more and more challenges as we grew. The incident that brought us to adulthood came in 2010 when Jonathan McPhee announced he was leaving. At the time we thought, 'Oh my God, what are we going to do?!' What happened to us felt like a tragedy, but we resolved to overcome it. And what did we do? We began talking to each other and listening to each other and coming up with our own fabulous ideas on how to go forward. We learned to stand on our own two feet."

During the 2011-2012 season, the LSO welcomed a series of guest conductors for our concerts and hoped to choose one to succeed McPhee. After playing under the baton of one of these guests in September 2011, Tom Sheldon said, "What was interesting about the concert is that we played so well. We watched our conductor, of course, but we were listening to each other much better than we ever had in the past. In the past, everything had to be funneled through Jonathan because he was such a capable and such a towering figure. Now we are taking control more ourselves. It's a really interesting concept when you think about leadership in general."

Bill Kates offered his "hats off" to the tremendous energy the members of the orchestra put into reorganizing the LSO after McPhee's announced departure. "People spent untold hours of their own time on that. So many people are now involved in the governance. There is now a leadership group that works together, not just a narrow leadership of a few people."

Sheldon said, "It's a good plan, I believe, and it is our future."

A Three-Part Mission

What will that leadership group face in the coming years? With the departure of McPhee, a new era of the LSO is about to begin. A new music director will bring his or her own musical direction and musical tastes to the ensemble. But the true direction of the Longwood Symphony, and its continued commitment to Healing the Community through Music, is in the hands of the organization itself. As I see it, our familiar symphonic concerts will be just one of three parts of our mission, along with two others that will become increasingly important: Community Engagement and Education.

"Community Engagement" refers to LSO on Call, our program that sends chamber groups of young doctors and medical students into hospitals and hospices and rehab centers. Goldstein said, "I'd like to see more of community connection, not just a hospital connection," and indeed that is what is beginning to really take root. While some of our performances are on hospital wards, many of them are in local senior centers, suburban hospices, and local Alzheimer's units. The musicians of the LSO jump at the chance to play in small ensembles at these medical facilities. Studying the impact of chamber music on Alzheimer's patients and senior citizens, their families, and their caregivers has the potential of changing the way we care for our aging population. We hope to expand our understanding of the neuroscience of music and how it can diminish pain and reduce the need for anesthesia and sedation, as discussed in Chapter Six.

Then there is our Educational work. Our symposia have brought colleagues from across the country and beyond to consider the fascinating and heady intersection between the arts and sciences. As described in Mannes' recent book, *The Power of Music*, the fields of the neuroscience of music and the neuroscience of healing are garnering great interest, thanks to new imaging techniques such as functional MRI and PET scanning. What impact and changes will this new knowledge have on how we combine music, medicine, and healing? How might it change the way we educate our music students? Our medical students? The Longwood Symphony Orchestra and its sister organizations around the country are well positioned to consider these options.

On a local level, the LSO can also become an advocate for musical education at the earliest level. Denise Lotufo is concerned that when schools face budget constraints, music is one of the first programs to get cut. "We have kids growing up who don't know what a violin sounds like. They may never have heard an acoustical musical instrument played in their presence. I'd like to see the LSO fill that niche."

My vision is that all three parts become equal at the Longwood Symphony Orchestra: the symphonic concerts, the community outreach, and the educational programs. The universal interest in music and its role in healing will continue to increase. For the past century we've put all our faith in technology, and now we're realizing its limits. We're coming back to what tradition has taught: examining our patients one on one, measuring their vital signs with our own eyes and ears, and determining courses of treatment based on hearing a heartbeat, feeling a forehead, peering into a throat. And truly listening to our patients. Our musical training helps us to listen, not just hear, and to recognize the melody behind the rote diagnosis.

Looking ahead, I feel that the fields of music education, music for healing, and music for social justice are intersecting. In this book we have met neuroscientists interested in the neuroimaging evidence of the permanent impact music has on the developing brain. There are other neuroscientists who are similarly investigating the impact of meditation, empathy, and altruism. It is likely that we will see these fields overlap, and the discovery that mindfulness, meditation, and music make healthy changes to the brain in similar areas. We already know that early music exposure positively impacts neural function and brain growth, including executive function; and we have seen how kids involved in music demonstrate enhanced creativity, discipline, and focus.

The field continues to grow and institutional lines continue to be crossed. Over the past few years, I have been excited to see that medical schools across the country are seeking each other out to jointly consider how the arts and humanities can be reincorporated into their curriculum. The work of the El Sistema movement here in the United States, from El Sistema USA to the New England Conservatory's Abreu Fellowship to the Los Angeles Philharmonic's Youth Orchestra of LA program, continues to gather momentum. Along with other game-changing programs, such as Providence, Rhode Island's Community MusicWorks that consider the role of music in the community and music for social change, a national rethinking of music curriculum may be on the horizon. Music education should no longer be viewed as an expendable separate entity in schools, but incorporated into language arts and social and natural sciences.

Music in the community is, in effect, preventive medicine. We can see this on the micro level—where music played by Longwood Symphony musicians for patients results in measurable changes in health. And we can see it on the macro level with our Healing Art of Music program and with El Sistema-inspired programs. Music goes a long way to heal entire communities. Social justice and social welfare are important determinants of health. Programs that look beyond the music are truly "Healing the Community through Music."

The growing body of evidence documenting the impact of music on the young brain and the success of programs like El Sistema make me hopeful that the relentless cutting of music, art, and humanities programs in our schools will reverse itself. Many of the musicians of the Longwood Symphony Orchestra were first exposed to music through their public schools, like Terry Buchmiller and Denise Lotufo. The

Longwood Symphony Orchestra, and other orchestras like it, have the responsibility to continue to move the conversation forward. We are living examples of why music education is important—not only because we became musicians, but because as musicians we have learned to embrace other healing careers. We know what a tremendous difference music in a life can make. Our biannual symposia "Crossing the Corpus Callosum" bring therapists, neuroscientists, and musicians together to discuss the healing arts of music and medicine. Over time, I hope this conversation extends to include leaders in the social services and education as well.

Mentoring Kids

In addition to playing and healing, a lot of us fulfill our educational urge in a very basic one-on-one way: we teach. This brings us into close contact with the next generation, and we give a lot of thought to what we impart to them. One model is provided by Dr. Tom Sheldon and Anand Jagannath, a young violinist with a big humanitarian heart who is a first-year medical student at Tufts. In 2010 Dr. Sheldon chaired the LSO's spirited Membership Task Force committee to explore the questions around what it means to be a member of the LSO and how to define that. One suggestion was that a way should be found for older doctors to partner with younger doctors in more formal mentorships. The LSO hosted a dinnertime soiree so they could meet and talk outside of rehearsals. He and Jagannath met at a Boston Symphony concert and Sheldon has taken the younger man under his wing.

"Anand was a sub for the LSO at the time, and as a regular member I barely knew the subs existed because we don't usually use them in the oboe section," Dr. Sheldon said. "I learned from him that it's very common for younger members to feel disenfranchised, like they don't really belong and aren't really sure where they fit in. These feelings start in middle school where there are a lot of cliques, but they sometimes persist into adulthood. There is a lot of anxiety about that. So one of the themes of our member task force became: how do we make people feel like they belong? Medicine is very complex and as you get older you do have a much broader view of things and so, from that standpoint, you feel like you have something to offer these younger players."

As for the orchestra as a whole, Sheldon said he believes the LSO will continue to attract musician-physicians as long as there is an audience for classical music. But he agrees that it depends a lot on how future generations are educated. "If they kill childhood musical education, then we are going to have a problem. But as long as some of the brightest people are trained in music when they are young, they will continue to want to be part of something like the LSO."

Sheldon's colleague, our young concertmaster Sherman Jia, said that his vision for the future of the LSO includes systematizing and formalizing mentorships like Dr. Sheldon's with medical student Anand Jagannath. His idea of forming Big Brother/Big Sister relationships between LSO members and young musician-physicians still in medical school is a great one. So many medical students are taught to suppress or ignore their musical abilities during medical training rather than to celebrate it and develop it as part of what Bill Kates calls "their medical selves."

And the mentoring could go both ways. "In medicine I'm the old guy, I'm the mentor," said Sheldon. "But now, someone like oboist Michael Barnett shows up and he's this fabulous multi-talented kid, and suddenly, musically, he's *my* mentor."

Can music gain a more active role in the training of doctors? While we've looked at studies that document the impact of music on patients, much work is left to be done to study the impact of music on the caregiver and on the caregiver/musician. Longitudinal studies of how playing music in healthcare settings changes the way a young medical student cares for his patient are waiting to be done. Perhaps they could point the way toward the humanities-in-medicine training that is on our horizon.

Mentoring Orchestras

Mentoring individual doctors and individual musicians has long been our goal. But several of our members envision an even bigger calling in our future: mentoring whole musician-physician orchestras.

Barnett said he would like to see the LSO reach out to other musician-physician groups across the U.S. and even internationally—not only showing them how we have solved our problems of how to pick the right conductors and build a repertoire with the right kinds of music, but also such nuts-and-bolts problems as publicity, administration, and financing. The story of the LSO's tenfold increase in budget over three decades could serve as an object lesson to those groups just beginning on that path. Barnett feels that over the next five years, 2012 to 2017, the LSO could begin hosting national conferences in Boston for existing musician-physician groups, and to take a leadership role in helping groups of musically inclined doctors to form new orchestras.

Such conferences "would help us to have a unified presence. We could use our talents as health professionals and musicians to show communities how to come together. Mature stability for us as an organization will give us the opportunity perhaps to make the world a little better place."

As an all-volunteer orchestra, we can focus on philanthropy because we don't have to struggle to find ways to pay the salaries of a hundred musicians, as most professional orchestras do. We pride ourselves on our amateur status. But perhaps we don't give ourselves enough credit.

Dr. Sheldon is a sociable man who often goes out with guests after concerts to get their feedback. He shared two comments that he felt had special resonance for us. "I once went out with friends from the American Cancer Society and one said that the LSO is perhaps the greatest collection of overachievers on one stage ever, and I think there's a lot of truth to that. Another time I went out with two of our guest soloists—these are professional musicians—and I asked them how they felt about playing with an amateur orchestra. One of them said, 'I don't know what exactly you are—but you're not amateurs.'

GROWING MINDFULLY

As we come to the end of this account, I'd like to turn now to the eldest person quoted in this book, Nobel Prize-winner (and LSO subscriber) Dr. Bernard Lown; and one of the youngest, Andrea Spencer.

The future will be in the hands of a new generation, people who are now musical students or residents. People like Spencer, the resident in psychiatry at Mass General and McLean Hospital, who has played viola for us since 2004. "I love this orchestra so much. When I came to Boston, the LSO was the only place I felt comfortable, so the question of what the orchestra will become in the next twenty-five years is one I'm very mindful of. As any organization grows, there is bound to be conflict. You saw what happened to our founders. They had to leave because of disputes, and it's naively optimistic to say that won't happen again. My sense right now is to take a step back and let it grow mindfully from here. If we put our minds to it, we will have the resilience to get through the growing pains in a way other organizations do not.

"For one thing," she said, "I'd like to see us build a network with other doctors' orchestras around the world, and find a way to help new such organizations get off the ground. I'm hoping LSO on Call will grow in its role and become an even stronger presence. Our sub list has grown so long we barely have room on that, let alone room in the orchestra. Involving those musicians in LSO on Call will create a way for us to engage our community in an even greater way. Everyone loves the LSO, and as long as that love continues, the LSO will continue."

The LSO can be, as Michael Barnett and Andrea Spencer envisioned, a convener for orchestras like it around the world, both those made up of musicians from the medical professions and those made up of musicians who simply want to devote their time making the world a better place. The goal is to make music part of a triumvirate with service and healing.

And to make them inextricably linked together, as they are in the LSO.

Medical schools, from Harvard to Stanford to Dalhousie in Nova Scotia, are spending increasing time on thinking about how to reintegrate the humanities into medical practice. How does one teach empathy to the technically trained young medical students? Through the arts. There are courses now that help young medical students realize that some of the challenges and horrors that they experience during their rigorous training cannot be expressed through words but can be expressed through the arts.

The work of people like Dr. Sandra Bertman, who has encouraged first-year medical students to create art to express their feelings about their first encounter with a cadaver as they learn Anatomy in their first year, and the work of Dr. Elizabeth Gaufberg, who teaches third-year medical students to break down their biases in observation through looking at contemporary art then reapplying it to their diagnostic skills, are just a tip of the iceberg.

At the same time, music schools are also scrutinizing the way they are training their students. From Juilliard to the New England Conservatory and beyond, these thoughtful faculty are considering ways to keep the humanism in music. They are offering courses in music and healing, as well as musical entrepreneurship and community engagement. Up to this time the music schools had focused primarily on helping the young musician hone his or her technical skill for their own professional careers. But in these times, as Jesse Rosen, president of the League of American Orchestras, has said, "Excellence is not enough. The orchestras and arts organizations of tomorrow need to meet the community where it is now." And engagement with the wider public will help cement a love for music and the other arts with a whole new generation.

Audiences now have more opportunities to see art forms that are different, engaging and life-sustaining in different ways. The days when there was a steady audience for Mahler alone are gone. Now the average audience member will choose to attend a rock concert on one night, an experiential drama on another, and a symphonic concert on another day.

Young musicians in the Longwood Symphony can observe firsthand what impact their musical performance has made on a patient dying of cancer or a dementia patient who can remember the words to a song from the 1940s but can't remember what she had for dinner. They can stop to realize that their hands-on musical therapy has touched their own hearts as well.

Dr. Lown looks at the efforts of the LSO as part of a very big picture. "I think we are coming to the end of a big historic period," he said. "I think we need a second Renaissance in which we begin to restore human connectivity. Instead of exchanging goods, we will exchange ideas and art and, yes, music. When you have an apple and I have an orange and we exchange them, we each still have only one fruit. But if I have an idea and you have an idea and we exchange them, then we both have two ideas, and that sparks something new, so you can sometimes get four or five from just one initial 'exchange.' That's the beauty of it. We need to restructure society around the exchange of art and ideas. The Longwood Symphony, through its devotion to music and to community service, is already advancing something like this idea."

CODA

When I joined the Longwood Symphony Orchestra in 1985, the group was barely two years old. We were an enthusiastic but rather motley band of eighty or ninety musicians, conducted by a young conductor who had just graduated from the New England Conservatory. But we set out some ambitious and lasting goals—to play orchestral music, in Jordan Hall. Soon we added to it an annual concert on the Esplanade. Our budget has grown from $33,000 to $300,000 and our Healing Art of Music program has raised nearly $1 million for the medically underserved. That is an amazing achievement for any organization, much less an orchestra!

After twenty seasons, I will be stepping down in 2012 as president of the LSO. As Denise Lotufo said, the LSO is a young adult, ready to leave the nest and take wing. With increased engagement by many, the future lies in the hands of the entire orchestra and board.

The future of our orchestra is bright and the possibilities are unlimited. The Longwood Symphony Orchestra will proudly continue its role as convener, catalyst, and mentor, and serve as an example of how music, medicine, and service can truly change the community I have great confidence that the LSO will fly farther and for longer than we ever thought possible twenty years ago.

Dr. Albert Schweitzer encourages us to "find your own Lambaréné," to find one's own way to serve. Like Dr. Schweitzer, the LSO has found its own unique way to serve, by combining music, medicine, and community service right here in Boston. The city—with all its wealth and poverty; its great institutions of culture, education, and medicine next to sinks of ignorance and violence—but above all the creative soul and the affluence of spirit that unites us as artists and scientists—*is* Longwood Symphony's very own Lambaréné.

Appendix A:
What We Listen To

Fans of the LSO often ask our members to name a few of their favorite pieces of music, to specify what kinds of music are best for different moods and situations, and to share what music we use to promote our own well-being. I've polled our musician-physicians and assembled this master playlist. The reader will likely think of others that should or could be on the list—please consider this a jumping off point for a lifetime of musical enjoyment and healing!

Suggested Favorite Works for Listening

BACH SONATAS AND PARTITAS FOR SOLO VIOLIN
Bach	"Goldberg Variations," BWV 988
Beethoven	Piano Concerto No. 4 in G major
Beethoven	All Beethoven Symphonies

Borodin	Il Notturno
Brahms	Clarinet Quintet
Brahms	A German Requiem, To Words of the Holy Scriptures, Op. 45
Brahms	String Quintet in G major, Op. 111
Brahms	Symphony No. 4 in E Minor, Op. 98
Corelli	Concerto Grosso in G Minor, Op. 6, No. 8, "Christmas" Concerto
Dvorak	String Quartet in F Major, Op. 96, "American" Quartet
Elgar	Variations on an Original Theme for orchestra ("Enigma"), Op. 36
Gershwin	Rhapsody in Blue
Mahler	Symphony No. 9
Mozart	Quintet for Clarinet and Strings, K. 581
Mozart	Sinfonia Concertante for Violin, Viola and Orchestra in E-flat Major, K. 364
Mozart	Piano Concerto No. 20 in D Minor, K. 466
Mozart	Piano Concerto No. 21 in C Major, K. 467
Mozart	Requiem Mass in D Minor
Rachmaninoff	Piano Concerto No. 2 in C Minor, Op. 18
Rachmaninoff	Symphonic Dances, Op. 45
Shostakovich	String Quartet No. 8 in C Minor, Op. 110
Sibelius	Violin Concerto in D Minor, Op. 47
Strauss	The Four Last Songs
Tchaikovsky	Music from Swan Lake, Op. 20

FAVORITE MUSIC TO PLAY

Elgar	Variations on an Original Theme for orchestra ("Enigma"), Op. 36

	Anything by Beethoven
	Anything by Mahler
Schubert	String Quintet in C Major, D. 956
Shostakovich	String Quartet No. 8 in C Minor, Op. 110
Shostakovich	Symphony No. 5 in D Minor, Op. 47

MUSIC FOR HEALING

Bach	Six Suites for Unaccompanied Cello
Barber	Adagio for Strings, Op. 11
Barber	Violin Concerto, Op. 14
Brahms	String Sextet in G Major, Op. 36
Haydn	The "Sun Quartets," Op. 20
Mozart	String Quintet in G Minor, K. 516
Mozart	Requiem Mass in D Minor
Ravel	Pavane for a Dead Princess
Rimsky-Korsakoff	from Scheherazade, Op. 35
Tchaikovsky	Serenade for Strings in C Major, Op. 48
Vaughan Williams	The Lark Ascending
Vaughan Williams	Mass in G Minor

MUSIC FOR STRESS RELIEF

Barber	Violin Concerto, Op. 14
Beethoven	Symphony No. 6 "Pastoral" in F Major, Op. 68
Corelli	Trio Sonata, Op. 1
Dvorak	String Quartet in F Major, Op. 96, "American" Quartet
Mahler	Symphony No. 5 in C-sharp Minor (Adagietto)

Mozart	Clarinet Concerto in A Major, K. 622
Rimsky-	
Korsakoff	Scheherazade, Op. 35
Schumann	Fantasie in C Major, Op. 17

MUSIC FOR PROBLEM SOLVING

Bach	The Concerto for 2 Violins, Strings and Continuo in D Minor, BWV 1043
Bach	"Goldberg Variations" BWV 988
Bach	"Italian" Concerto BWV 971
Brahms	Piano Concerto No. 1 in D minor, Op. 15
Brahms	Piano Concerto No. 2 in B-flat major, Op. 83
Liszt	Totentanz, S. 126
Monteverdi	Vespers of 1610

MUSIC FOR DEEP EMOTIONS

Beethoven	Symphony No. 3, "Eroica" in E-flat Major, Op. 55
Beethoven	Violin Concerto in D major, Op. 61
Bernstein	Symphony No. 1, "Jeremiah"
Brahms	A German Requiem, To Words of the Holy Scriptures, Op. 45
Brahms	String Sextet in B-flat Major, Op. 18
Mahler	Symphony No. 1
Mahler	Symphony No. 10
Schubert	String Quintet in C Major, D. 956
Shostakovich	String Quartet No. 8 in C Minor, Op. 110
Vaughan Williams	"A Sea Symphony"

MUSIC FOR COMMUNITY

Bach   The Concerto for 2 Violins, Strings and
Continuo in D Minor, BWV 1043
Vivaldi   "The Four Seasons"
Haydn   "The Creation"
Anything by John Philip Sousa
Vaughan Williams Piano Quintet in C Minor

JUST FOR FUN

Antonio Bazzini   Dance of the Goblins

Appendix B:
Personal Suggestions from the
Musician-Physicians

TERRY BUCHMILLER

Beethoven's Ninth Symphony, particularly the last movement. It's a gigantic musical essay on the human condition. When the choir lets out the "Ode to Joy," I think the clouds part! Also, if I can complete a 5K run while listening to this movement, I know I'm doing OK! Beethoven's Seventh Symphony was one of the first pieces I played in Youth Symphony. I especially loved the slow movement. I think it helped provide a transition from grade school technician to a musician who was part of a larger whole. It was such a connection! And Barber's "Adagio for Strings" is etherial: life, angst, death . . . and life again.

HEIDI HARBISON KIMBERLY

I love Bach's unaccompanied cello suites, preferably played by Yo-Yo Ma. My friend from college played the Suite No. 1 at our wedding. Imagine listening to Bach played outside on a beautiful day atop a hill overlooking a lake! I also have a wonderful association with that piece since it is one of my Dad's favorite pieces to practice on his viola—in the kitchen because it had the best (and loudest) acoustics in the house.

I also love Bach's unaccompanied violin sonatas and partitas. They are meditative, simple, and stunning. When I want to just play music and not practice, I get lost in a Bach unaccompanied sonata or partita. I brought a violin when I was trekking through the Himalayas in Nepal and played Bach outside, in the shadow of the Annapurna. I also loved watching the video of Joshua Bell playing the Bach "Chaconne" in the DC subway station.

I would also recommend Brahms' symphonies (all of them) and Brahms' sextets (both of them), and the Schubert Cello Quintet. It has one of my all-time favorite melodies. There is a great documentary about the Philadelphia Orchestra called Music From the Inside Out in which the concertmaster calls the Schubert Cello Quintet "pure ecstasy."

One more thing: Rachmaninoff's Symphonic Dances. On one of the hottest days of the summer I made my kids sit in the car after we got to the pool so we could finish listening to the saxophone solo from this.

DANIELA KRAUSE

My favourite pieces of music are anything by Gustav Mahler. All his work are such deep reflections of his personal biography, just as if he composed in order to heal himself. Any kind of classical music really has "healing power" for me. There are fine nuances in every piece.

Psyche Loui

I am particularly attracted to music that gives me physiological reactions such as chills/goosebumps, makes me tear up, or gives me a feeling in the pit of my stomach. Some of these pieces include the Rachmaninoff Second Piano Concerto (second movement), Mozart's Piano Concerto No. 20 (second movement), and Brahms Symphony No. 1 (first movement). The Mozart in particular has a healing effect, I think.

Peter Stein

I'm a sucker for any music that, without sentimentality, traces a course from darkness to light, despair to joy, hurt to healing. That takes in quite a lot of music! But a short, idiosyncratic list would include Brahms' "German Requiem" and, on the chamber music side, his second String Quintet and String Sextet (both in G major); and Bach's B-minor Mass. Mozart's G-minor String Quintet (K.516) is another example, one of the most penetrating musical testimonies of bitterness and happiness I can think of. Of course this is also one of the major themes in Beethoven's work, and he left us too many examples to cite! But to me, life would be poorer without his Seventh Symphony. The Ninth is a more obvious example, but it's the Seventh that leaves me healed.

Music for a Wedding—Lisa Wong

When Lynn and I were married, we chose music for a piano quartet consisting of dear friends Daniel Phillips, Michael Stern, Yo-Yo Ma and Luise Vosgerchian. The wedding opened with the slow movement of Mozart's Piano Quartet in g minor. The processional was the Andante from Brahms' 3rd piano Quartet in c minor. In lieu of a homily, we all sat to listen to Schumann's beautiful Andante Cantabile from his Piano Quartet in Eb major and recessed out to the last movement, Vivace. The beauty of the cello solos and rich harmonies of the strings and piano still ring in my ear.

Works Cited

Bertman, Sandra L. *Grief and the Healing Arts: Creativity as Therapy.* Amityville, NY: Baywood Pub., 1999. Print.

Bornstein, David. *How to Change the World.* Oxford: Oxford UP, 2007. Print.

Boyer, Johanna Misey. *Creativity Matters: The Arts and Aging Toolkit.* New York, NY: National Guild of Community Schools of the Arts, 2007. Print.

Callahan, Suzanne. *Singing Our Praises: Case Studies in the Art of Evaluation.* [S.l.]: Assoc of Performing Arts, 2006. Print.

Eagleman, David. *Incognito: The Secret Lives of the Brain.* New York: Pantheon, 2011. Print.

Harkleroad, Leon. *The Math Behind the Music.* Cambridge: Cambridge UP, 2006. Print.

Hartley, Nigel, and Malcolm Payne. *The Creative Arts in Palliative Care*. London: Jessica Kingsley, 2008. Print.

Huron, David. *Sweet Anticipation*. Cambridge: MIT, 2007. Print.

Langer, Ellen J. *On Becoming an Artist: Reinventing Yourself through Mindful Creativity*. New York: Ballantine, 2005. Print.

Lehrer, Jonah. *Proust Was a Neuroscientist*. Boston: Houghton Mifflin, 2007. Print.

Levitin, Daniel J. *The World in Six Songs: How the Musical Brain Created Human Nature*. New York: Dutton, 2008. Print.

Levitin, Daniel J. *This Is Your Brain on Music: The Science of a Human Obsession*. New York, NY: Dutton, 2006. Print.

Lown, B. *The Lost Art of Healing*. Boston: Houghton Mifflin, 1996. Print.

Mannes, Elena. *The Power of Music: Pioneering Discoveries in the New Science of Song*. New York: Walker &, 2011. Print.

May, Elizabeth. *Musics of Many Cultures: An Introduction*. Berkeley: University of California, 1980. Print.

McNiff, Shaun. *Art as Medicine: Creating a Therapy of the Imagination*. Boston: Shambhala, 1992. Print.

Neumayr, Anton, and David J. Parent. *Music and Medicine: Chopin, Smetana, Tchaikovsky, Mahler: Notes on Their Lives, Works, and Medical Histories*. Print.

Neumayr, Anton. *Music and Medicine*. Bloomington, IL: Medi-Ed, 1994. Print.

Patel, Aniruddh D. *Music, Language, and the Brain*. Oxford: Oxford UP, 2008. Print.

Sacks, Oliver W. *Musicophilia: Tales of Music and the Brain*. New York: Alfred A. Knopf, 2007. Print.

Stravinsky, Igor, Arthur Knodel, and Ingolf Dahl. *Poetics of Music: In the Form of Six Lessons.* Cambridge: Harvard UP, 1947. Print.

Tepper, Steven J., and Bill J. Ivey. *Engaging Art: The next Great Transformation of America's Cultural Life.* New York: Routledge, 2008. Print.

Additional Articles

Al-Talbi, Ammar. "Al-Farabi." *Prospects: the Quarterly Review of Comparative Education* 23.1 (1993): pp. 353–372.

Amunts K., Schlaug G., Jancke L., Steinmetz H., Dabringhaus A., Zilles K., Schleicher A. "Motor Cortex and Hand Motor Skills: Structural Compliance in the Human Brain." *Human Brain Mapping* 5 (1997): pp. 206–215. Print.

Blood A., Zatorre R. "Intensely Pleasurable Responses to Music Correlate with Activity in Brain Regions Implicated in Reward and Emotion." *PNAS* 98.20 (2001): pp. 11818–11823.

Cepeda MS, Carr DB, Lau J, Alvarez H. "Music for pain relief (Review)." *The Cochrane Collaboration* 3 (2007).

Cerda JJ. "Art in Medicine: Musicians, Physicians and Physician-Musician." *Transactions of the American Clinical and Climatological Association* 104 (1993): pp. 228–234.

Cromer, Janet. "Creative Connections." Health Care, 10 July 2007. Boston.com.

Curtis ME, Bharucha JJ. "The Minor Third Communicates Sadness in Speech, Mirroring its Use in Music." *Emotion* 10.3 (2010): pp. 335–48.

Davidoff F. "Music Lessons: What Musicians Can Teach Doctors (and Other Health Professionals)." *Annals of Internal Medicine* 154.6 (2011): pp. 426–429.

Dissanayake, Ellen. Rev. of "The Singing Neanderthals: The Origins of Music, Language, Mind and Body" by Steven Mithen. <human-nature.com> 3 (2005): pp. 375–380.

Anders Ericsson, Michael Prietula, Edward Cokely. "The Making of an Expert." *The Harvard Business Review.* July 2007.

Evans HM. "Music, Medicine, and Embodiment." *The Lancet* 375.9718 (2010): pp. 886–887.

Gillespie WF. "Doctors and Music." *Canadian Medical Association Journal* 33.6 (1935): pp. 676–679.

Graves, Helen. "Adoptees From Korea Reach Across the Years and Miles Siblings via Adoption, Pair Take Separate Paths to Find Birth Families." *The Boston Globe.* 29 April. 2001.

Hanser SB. "From Ancient to Integrative Medicine, Models for Music Therapy." *Music and Medicine* 1.2 (2009): pp. 87–96.

Hyde KL., Lerch J., Norton A., Forgeard M., Winner E., Evans AC., Schlaug G. "Musical Training Shapes Structural Brain Development." *The Journal of Neuroscience* 29.10 (2009): pp. 3019–3025.

Jarvela, Irma. "Listening to Music is Biological." <eurkalert.org>, 25 February 2011.

Katz AM., Conant L., Inui TS., Baron David., Bor D. "A Council of Elders: Creating a Multi-Voiced Dialogue in a Community of Care." *Social Science and Medicine* 50.6 (2000): pp. 851–860.

Munte TF., Altenmuller E., Jancke L. "The Musician's Brain as a Model of Neuroplasticity." *Nature Reviews Neuroscience* 3 (2002): pp. 473–478.

Patel AD. "Language, Music, Syntax and the Brain." *Nature Neuroscience* 6.7 (2003): pp. 674–81.

Salamon, Maureen. "Laughter, Music May Lower Blood Pressure, Study Says." *Health Day.* 25 March. 2011.

Smyth J., Stone A., Hurewitz A., Kaell A. "Effects of Writing About Stressful Experiences on Symptom Reduction in Patients with Asthma or Rheumatoid Arthritis: a Randomized Trial." *JAMA* 281 (1999): pp. 1304–9.

Taylor DB. "Music in general hospital treatment from 1900 to 1950." *The Journal of Music Therapy* 18.2 (1981): pp. 62–73. Print.

Wang, Shirley. "Music Helps Stroke Victims Communicate, Study Finds." *The Wall Street Journal.* 22 February. 2010.

Wolf, Lea. "Music and Healthcare: A Paper Commissioned by the Musical Connections Program of Carnegie Hall's Weill Music Institute." Carnegie Hall and WolfBrown, August 2011.

"The Biology of Music." *The Economist.* 10 February 2000.

"Healing By Music Tried in Hospitals." *New York Times.* 20 March. 1938. ProQuest Historical Newspapers. *The New York Times* (1851–2007): 43.

"Music Therapy Interventions in Trauma, Depression, & Substance Abuse: Selected References and Key Findings." *American Music Therapy Association.* <www.musictherapy.org/assets/1/7/bib_mentalhealth.pdf>

Longwood Symphony Orchestra's Community Partners 1991–2011

Albert Schweitzer Fellowship
ALS Association Massachusetts Chapter
ALS Therapy Development Institute
American Epilepsy Society
Artists for Alzheimer's
Art in Giving—Rachel Molly Markoff Foundation
Asian Task Force Against Domestic Violence (ATASK)
Berkshire Children and Families
Boston Health Care for the Homeless Program
Boston Private Industry Council's School to Careers Program
Children of Chornobyl
Classical Action: Performing Arts Against AIDS
Dimock Community Health Center
Families of Spinal Muscular Atrophy

Friends of Brookline Public Health
Friends of LADDERS
Global Health Initiative at Boston University
Harvard Humanitarian Initiative at Harvard University
Harvard Medical School
Hospitality Homes
Japan Disaster Relief Fund—Boston
Joslin Diabetes Center
March of Dimes
Massachusetts League of Community Health Centers
Mattapan Community Health Center
New England Hemophilia Association
New England SERVE
Partners in Health
Performers' Outreach
Physicians for Human Rights
Project STEP
Reid Sacco Memorial Foundation
Seven Hills Behavioral Health
Sharing Foundation
Shriners Burn Hospital
St. Jude Children's Research Hospital
Steve Glidden Foundation
The Food Project
The Sharewood Project
Young Audiences of Massachusetts

Notes

CHAPTER 2

1. "The Edge of the Primeval Forest," Dr. Albert Schweitzer. Translator: C. T. Campion. AMS Press Inc. (Reprint of the 1948 edition published by Macmillan.)

CHAPTER 3

1. "What Would Hippocrates Do?" by Tara Parker-Pope, *New York Times* September 23, 2008.

2. "Making the 'Great Book of Songs': Compilation and the Author's Craft in Abû I-Faraj al-Isbahânî's Kitâb al-aghânî" by Hilary Kilpatrick. *Routledge Studies in Middle Eastern Literatures.*

3. *Prospects: the quarterly review of comparative education.* (Paris, UNESCO: International Bureau of Education), vol. XXIII, no. ½, 1993, pp. 353–372. ©UNESCO: International Bureau of Education, 2000. No author credited.

4. "Psychology from Islamic Perspective: Contributions of Early Muslim Scholars and Challenges to Contemporary Muslim Psychologists" by Amber Haque. Journal of Religion and Health 43 (4), 2004: pp. 357–377 [363].

5. "Philosophies of Music in Medieval Islam" by Fadlou Shehadi. *Brill's Studies in Intellectual History*, Leiden: E. J. Brill, 1995, p. 72.
6. "Borodin" by Sergei Aleksandrovich Dianin, Greenwood Press, 1980.
7. *Time Magazine*, June 4, 1934.
8. "Blue Gene Tyranny," All Music Guide.
9. "Stiff: The Curious Life of Human Cadavers," by March Roach. WW North & Co. p. 47.
10. "Little-Known Aspect of Theodor Billroth's Work: His Contribution to Musical Theory." *World Journal of Surgery*, Springer New York, Volume 21, Number 5 / June, 1997, pp. 569-571.
11 "Brahms and Billroth" by Daniel F. Roses, *The American Brahms Society Newsletter*, Volume V, Number 1, Spring 1987.
12. Letter to Lubke, quoted in F. William Sunderman, "Theodor Billroth as Musician", *Bulletin of the Medical Library Association*, 25/4, May 1937.
13. *The Independent*, April 23, 2001, obituary.
14. "Physician by Day, Musician by Night" by John Donvan and Christina Romano ABC News July 26, 2009.
15. "Eddie Henderson: Healing with Music" by R.J. De Luke. *All About Jazz*, undated.
16. Meyer, Marvin and Bergel, Kurt. *Reverence for Life: The Ethics of Albert Schweitzer for the Twenty-First Century*, p. 272.
17. The Nobel Foundation official biography, 1952 From Nobel Lectures, Peace 1951-1970, Editor Frederick W. Haberman, Elsevier Publishing Company, Amsterdam, 1972.
18. "Music in the Life of Albert Schweitzer: Selections from His Writings," by Charles R. Joy. London, A. & C. Black, 1953.
19. "Schweitzer, Albert, J.S. Bach," translated [into English] by Ernest Newman. 2 vols. London, A. & C. Black, 1911. (First published in French, J.S. Bach: Le Musicien-poète. Avec la collaboration de M. Hubert Gillot. Paris, Costallat, 1905.)
20. "Out of My Life and Thought: An Autobiography" ("Aus meinem Leben und Denken" by Albert Schweitzer. Leipzig, Felix Meiner, 1931.) Translated by C.T. Campion. New York, Henry Holt, 1933; 1949.

CHAPTER 5

1. "Music Helps Physicians Heal Themselves," National Public Radio's "Morning Edition," first broadcast November 15, 2004.

2. "HLA B*5701 is highly associated with restriction of virus replication in a subgroup of HIV-infected long-term nonprogressors" by Stephen A. Migueles, M. Shirin Sabbaghian, et al, "Proceedings of the National Academy of Science" USA March 14, 2000, 97 (6): 2709-2714.

3. "AIDS and the Secret of Long-Term Survivors" *The New York Times*, May 4, 2005. Posted on NYTimes.com website. No byline listed.

CHAPTER 6

1. "From Ancient to Integrative Medicine: Models for Music Therapy Music and Medicine" by Suzanne B. Hanser. *Music and Medicine*, Volume 1 Number 2. October 2009 87-96 # 2009. p. 87.

2. Ibid., p. 90.

3. "Music for Pain Relief" by G. Cepeda MS, Carr DB, Lau J, Alvarez H. *Cochrane Database of Systematic Reviews* 2006, Issue 2. Art. No.: CD004843. DOI: 10.1002/14651858.CD004843.pub2.

4. "Music in General Hospital Treatment from 1900 to 1950" by Dale B. Taylor, The University of Kansas. *Journal of Music Therapy* 1981, p. 62-83 54. ibid. (Vescelius 1918, p. 376).

5. Ibid.

6. *AMT Official History of Music Therapy*, no author cited.

7. "Music Therapy Helps Vets Control Symptoms of PTSD," by Abbie Fentress Swanson. WNYC.org, posted September 4, 2010.

8. "History of Music Therapy," no author cited. *Music as Medicine*, undated.

9. "Music Therapy Helps Vets Control Symptoms of PTSD," by Abbie Fentress Swanson. WNYC.org, posted September 4, 2010.

10. "Using Music To Manage PTSD Symptoms," no author cited. Disabilitylawclaims.com, posted September 9, 2010.

11. "Music Therapy Eases Post-Traumatic Stress Disorder for Families" by Kayla Turo. © 2011 *Making Music Magazine*.

12. "Music for Pain Relief," published in Cochrane Review by The Cochrane Collaboration in 2006.

13. "Intensely pleasurable responses to music correlate with activity in brain regions implicated in reward and emotion," by Anne J. Blood and Robert J. Zatorre .Montreal Neurological Institute, McGill University, Montreal, QC, Canada H3A 2B4 Edited by Marcus E. Raichle, Washington

University School of Medicine, St. Louis, MO, and approved July 16, 2001 (received for review July 11, 2001).

14. "The Role of the Premotor Cortex in Sensorimotor Transformations for Music Production," *Songs of Experience: Music and the Brain* by Joyce L. Chen, McGill University, Virginia B. Penhune, BRAMS, Concordia University, Montreal; and Robert J. Zatorre, BRAMS, McGill University, Montreal Neurological Institute. Presented at the Neurosciences and Music conferences, organized by the Mariani Foundation, with cooperation from the New York Academy of Sciences (NYAS). Al Convegno Internazionale "The Neurosciences and Music - II", Lipsia, 5-8 May 2005.

15. "Does Music Make You Exercise Harder?" by Gretchen Reynolds. Sc and J Med Sci Sports. Aug. 25, 2010;b20(4):662-9. Epub 2009 Sept. 28. Based on research paper "Effects of music tempo upon submaximal cycling performance" by Waterhouse J, Hudson P, Edwards B. Research Institute for Sport and Exercise Sciences, Liverpool John Moores University, Liverpool, U.K.

16. "Music Therapy Prepares Moms and Dads for Easier Childbirth," Health Magazine.

17. USA Today: "Music Provides Audio Analgesic" by Kim Painter. *USA Today*, July 10, 2006.

18. McDermott, K. (2001) "Music, Relaxation Can Complement Pain Medication, ScienceDaily.com, cited in *The Psychology of Music*, Suite101. com.

19. "Oregon cops hope classical music deters loiterers," by Nigel Duara. Associated Press, April 4, 2011.

20. "This Is Your Brain on Music: The Science of a Human Obsession," by Daniel J. Levitin, P 172.

21. Interview with Zyman, *Juilliard Journal*, undated.

CHAPTER 7

1. *Outliers: The Story of Success* by Malcolm Gladwell, Little, Brown and Company, 2008.

2. Harvard Business Review, July 2007, Ericsson, Prietula, Cokely.

3. "Musical Training Improves Your Children's Speech, Reading Vocabulary," by Professor Nina Kraus, "Nature Reviews Neuroscience," *Nature* magazine.

4. "Musical Training Shapes Structural Brain Development" by

Krista L. Hyde, Jason Lerch, Gottfried Schlaug, at al. *The Journal of Neuroscience*, 11 March 2009, 29(10): 3019-3025; doi: 10.1523/JNEUROSCI.5118-08.2009.

5. "No Einstein in Your Crib? Get a Refund" by Tamar Lewin, *New York Times*, Oct. 23, 2009.

6. "The musician's brain as a model of neuroplasticity" by Thomas F. Münte, Eckart Altenmüller and Lutz Jäncke in *Nature Reviews* Volume 3, June 2002, pp. 473-478.

7. "Motor Cortex and Hand Motor Skills: Structural Compliance in the Human Brain" by Katrin Amunts, Gottfried Schlaug, Lutz Jäncke, et al. *Human Brain Mapping*, 5:206–215, 1997. ©Wiley-Liss, Inc.

8. *The Power of Music: Pioneering Discoveries in the New Science of Song* by Elena Mannes, Walker & Company, 2011, pp. 42–43.

9. "Autism Spectrum Disorders: Music Therapy Research and Evidence-Based Practice Support" no byline. *American Music Therapy Association*, March 2, 2008.

10. Music Therapy for the Autistic Child by Juliette Alvin and Auriel Warwick. 1992 Oxford University Press, Edition: 2.

11. "Education: Music Therapy and Language" by Myra J. Staum, Ph.D., RMT-BC, National Association for Music Therapy, © 1967-2011 Autism Research Institute.

12. "Music in intervention for children and adolescents with Autism: A meta-analysis" by Jennifer Whipple. Journal of Music Therapy, Vol 41(2), Sum 2004, 90-106.

CHAPTER 8

1. "In Vivo Evidence of Structural Brain Assymetry in Musicians," Gottfried Schlaug, Lutz Jancke, Yanxiong Huang, Helmuth Steinmetz, in Science, vol. 267. February 2, 1995.

2. *This is your Brain on Music,* by Daniel J. Levitin (Plume/Penguin, 2007) pp. 124-125.

3. 'Formal Art Observation Training Improves Medical Students' Visual Diagnostic Skills" by Sheila Naghshineh, M.D., Janet P. Hafler, Ed.D., et al, in the Journal of General Internal Medicine, July 2008.

CHAPTER 9

1. Gray Matters: Music and the Brain, Public Radio International,

transcript at http://dana.org/dabi/transcripts/gm_0398.html. © 1998 The Charles A. Dana Foundation.

2. Riby DM, Hancock PJ (2008). "Viewing it differently: Social scene perception in Williams syndrome and Autism". Neuropsychologia 46 (11): 2855–60. doi:10.1016/j.neuropsychologia.2008.05.003. PMID 18561959.

3. Tomaino: http://www.caring.com/interviews/concetta-tomaino-about-music-therapy-for-alzheimer-s-patients.

CHAPTER 10

1. "Brain Structures Differ between Musicians and Non-Musicians" by Christian Gaser and Gottfried Schlaug, *The Journal of Neuroscience*, October 8, 2003.

CHAPTER 11

1. Aliment Pharmacol Ther. 2009 Oct;30(7):718-24. Epub 2009 Jul 8. El-Hassan H, McKeown K, Muller AF.

2. Music Therapy Studies Show Health Benefits, Therapy Times, 08.07.07.

3. "Music in Hospitals is Good Medicine for Anyone (But you don't have to have a malady to be healed by melody." Discovery.com/Planet Green.

4. "The Healing Power of Death Metal" Slate magazine, Anne Applebaum, Aug. 3, 2009.

CHAPTER 12

1. "Eddie Henderson: Healing With Music," *All About Jazz* 2011.

2. Rohter, Larry "Latin American Singer's Rainbow Coalition of Identities." *The New York Times*, July 12, 2005.